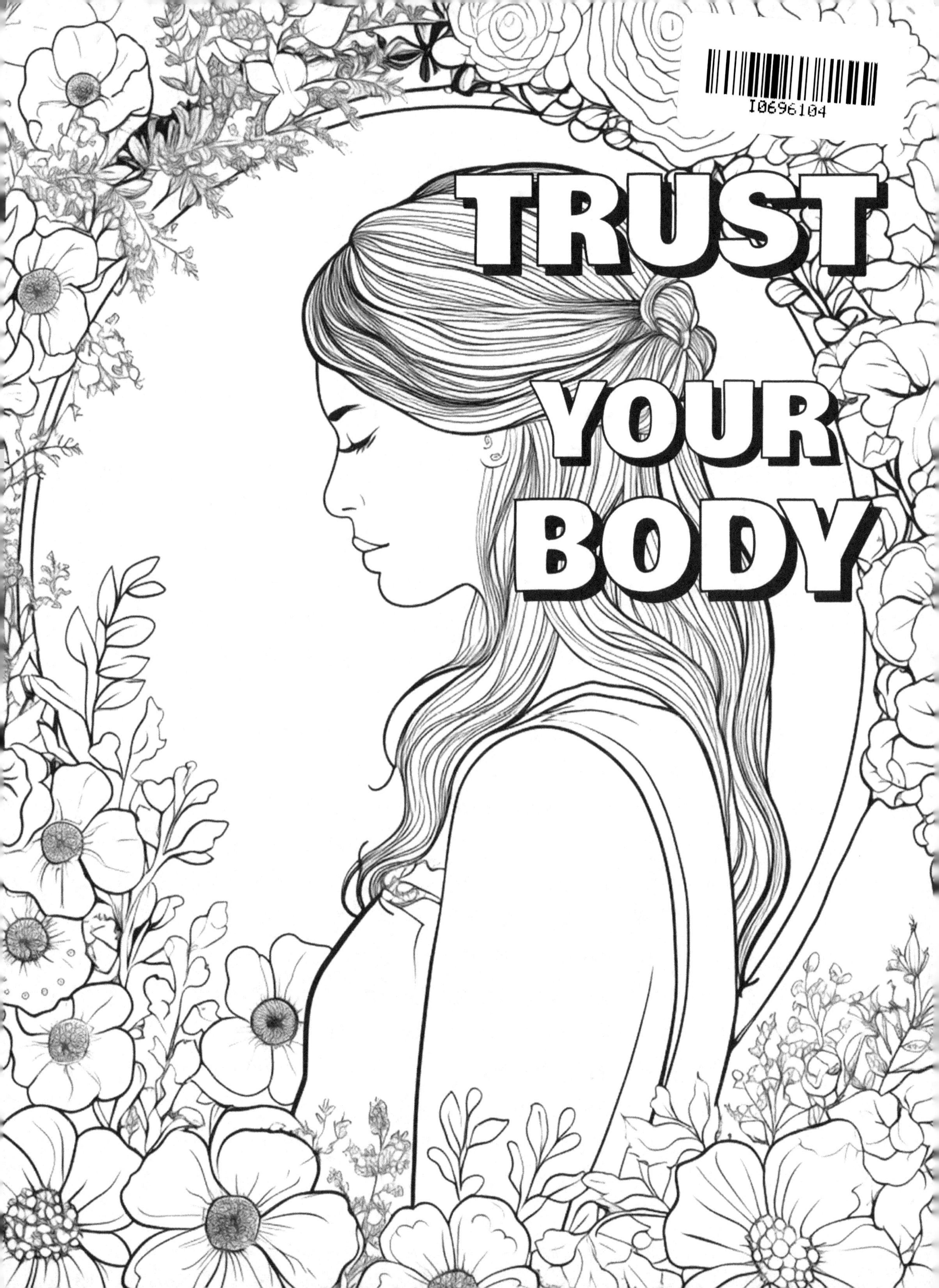

TRUST
YOUR
BODY

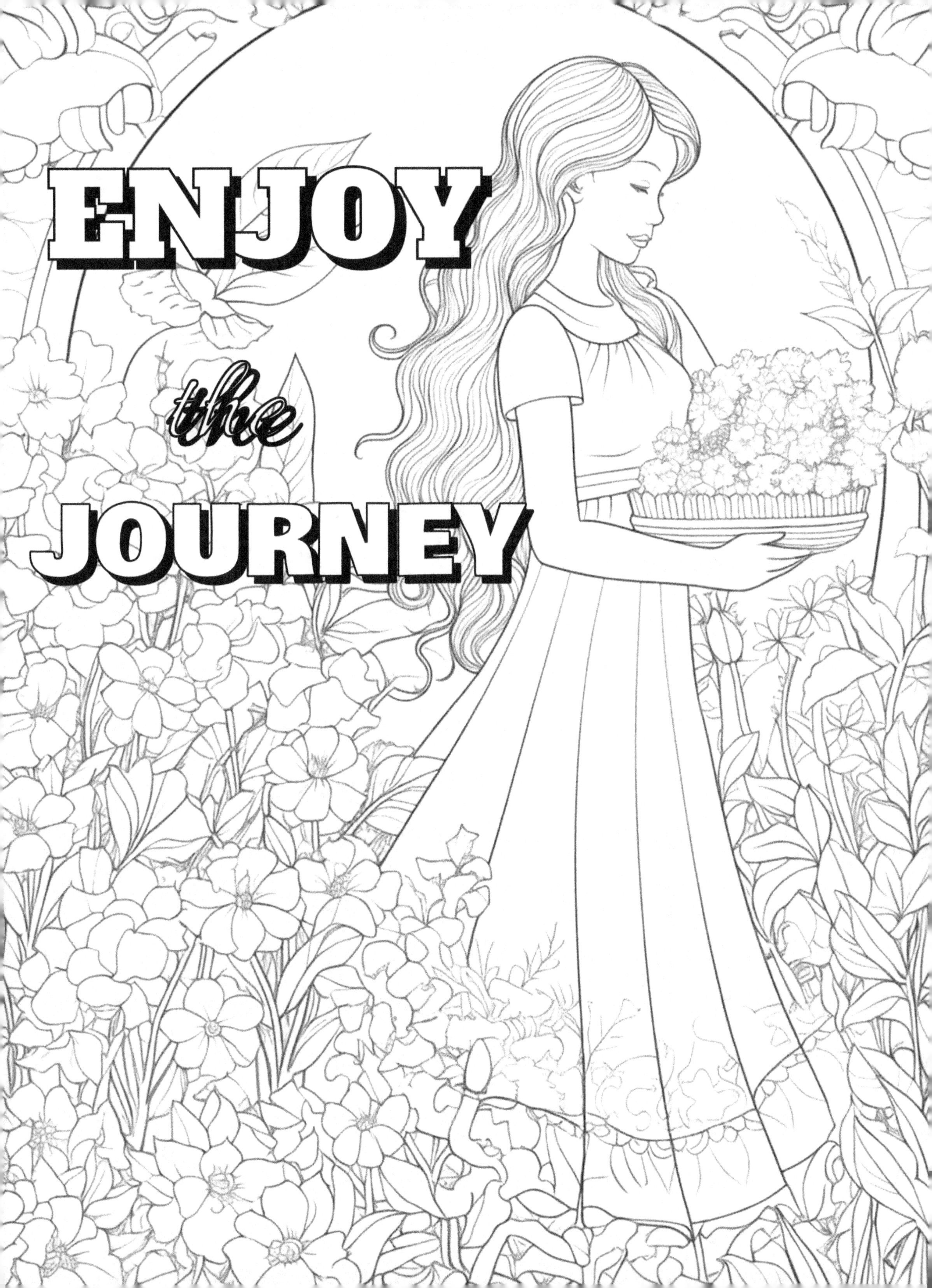

ENJOY
the
JOURNEY

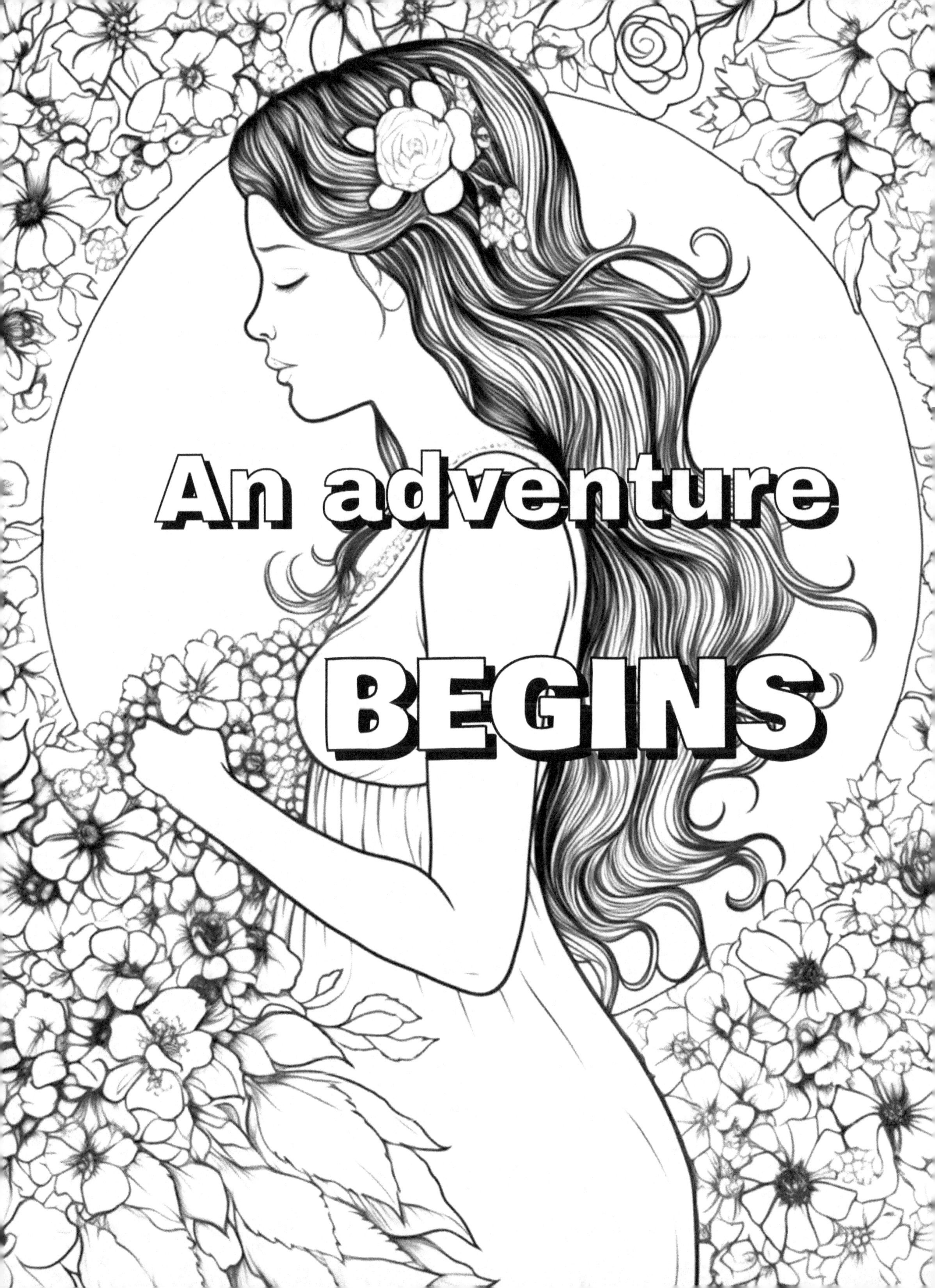

An adventure
BEGINS

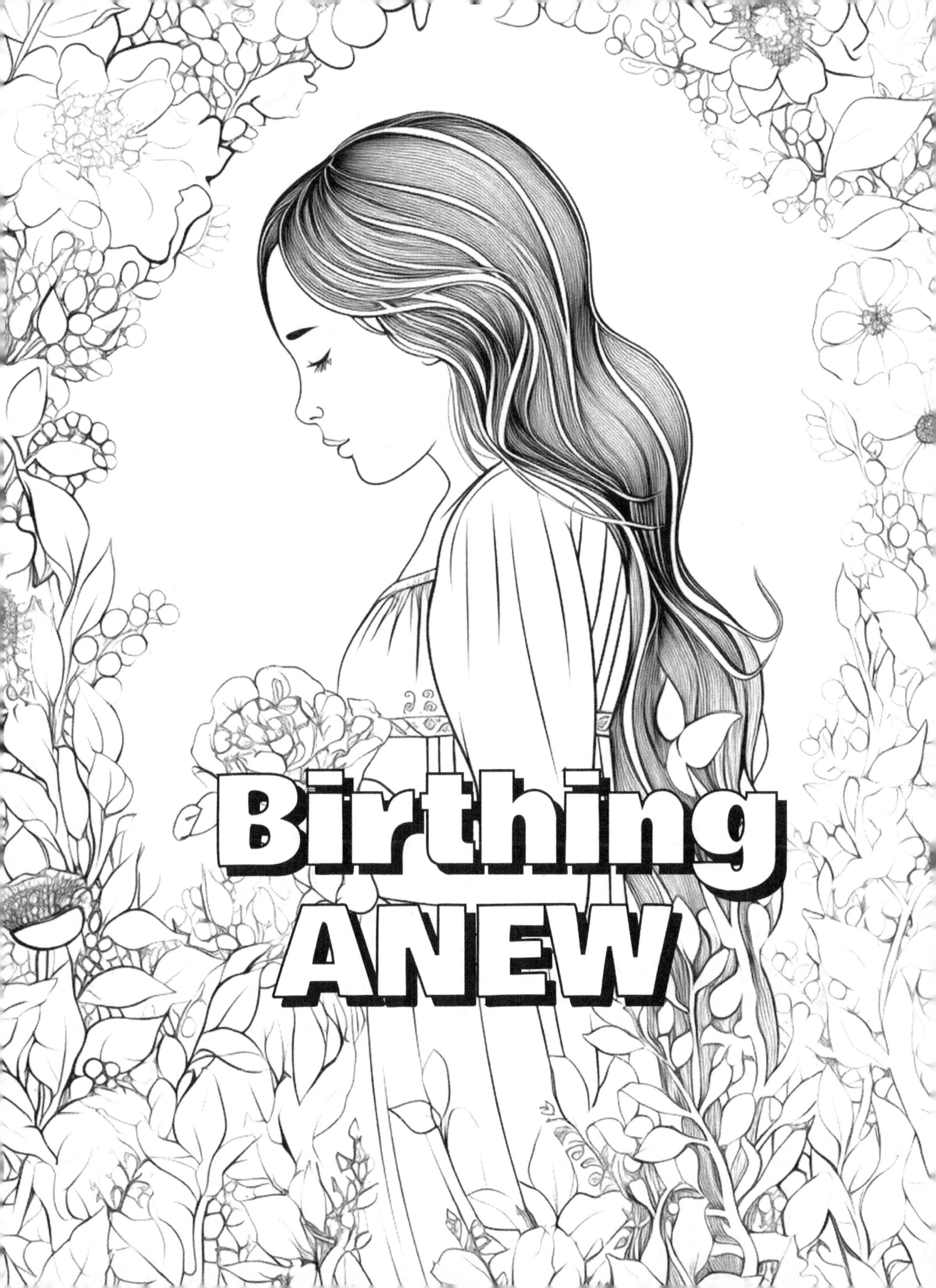

Birthing
ANEW

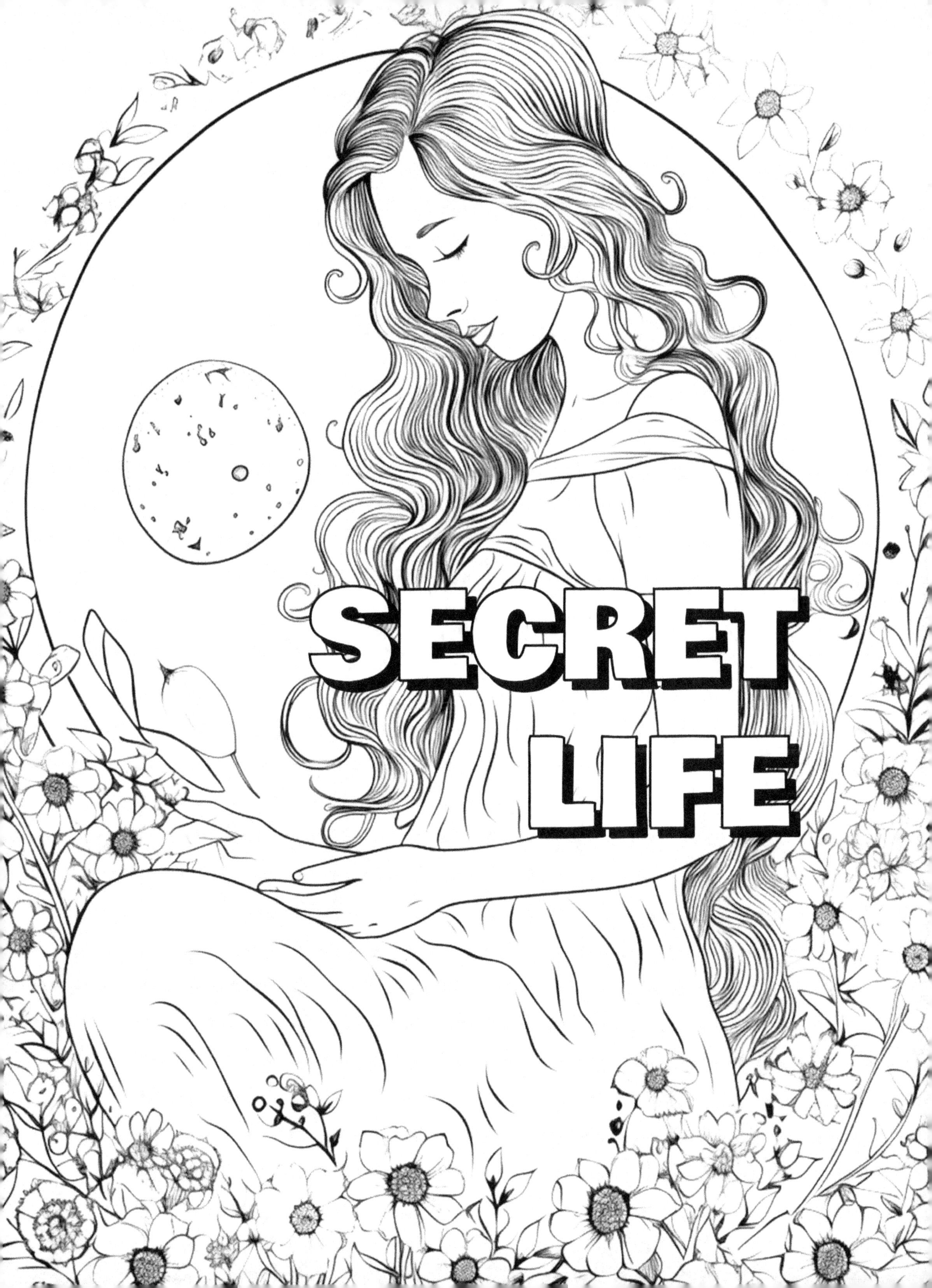

SECRET
LIFE

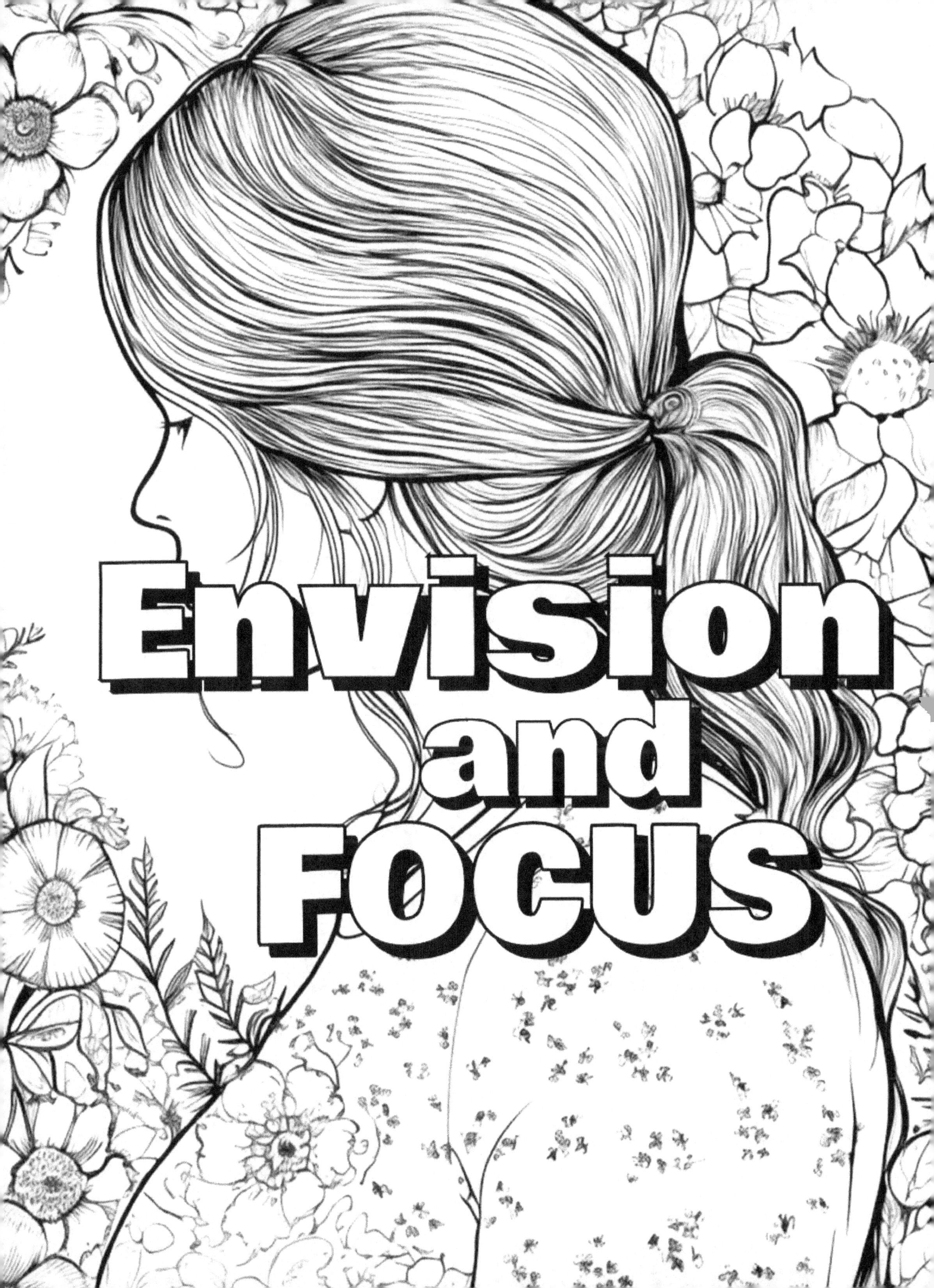
Envision
and
FOCUS

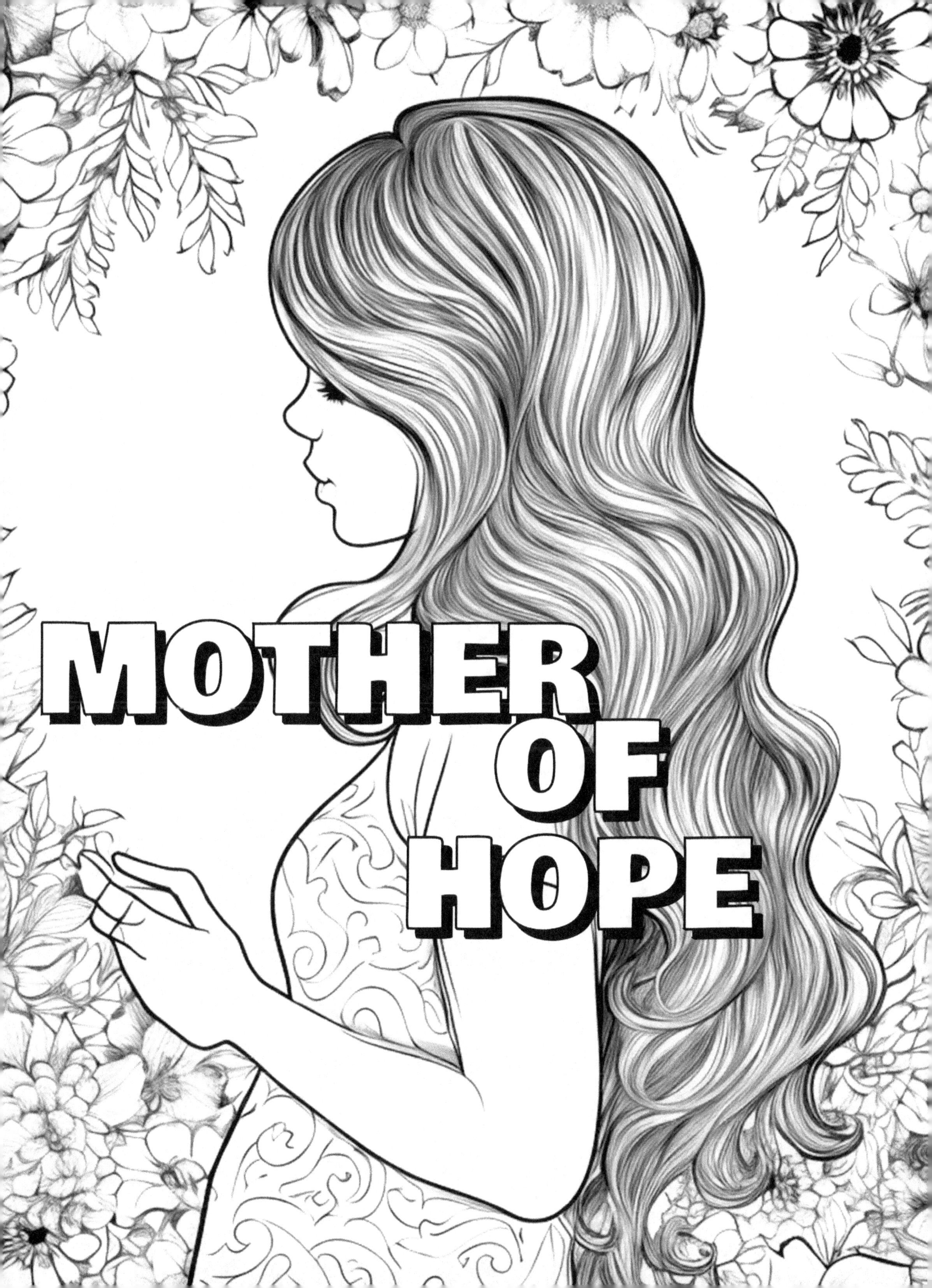

MOTHER
OF
HOPE

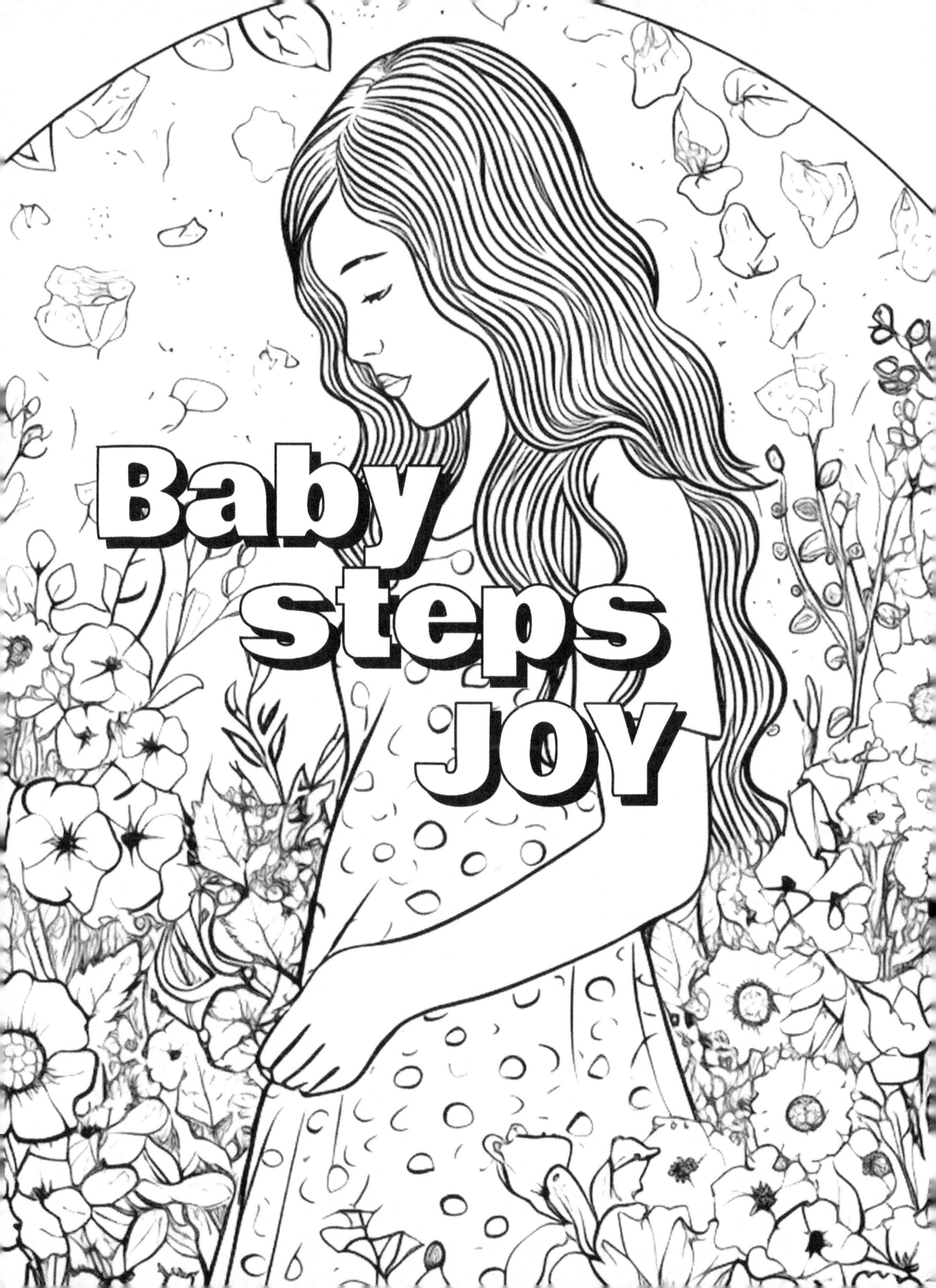
Baby
steps
JOY

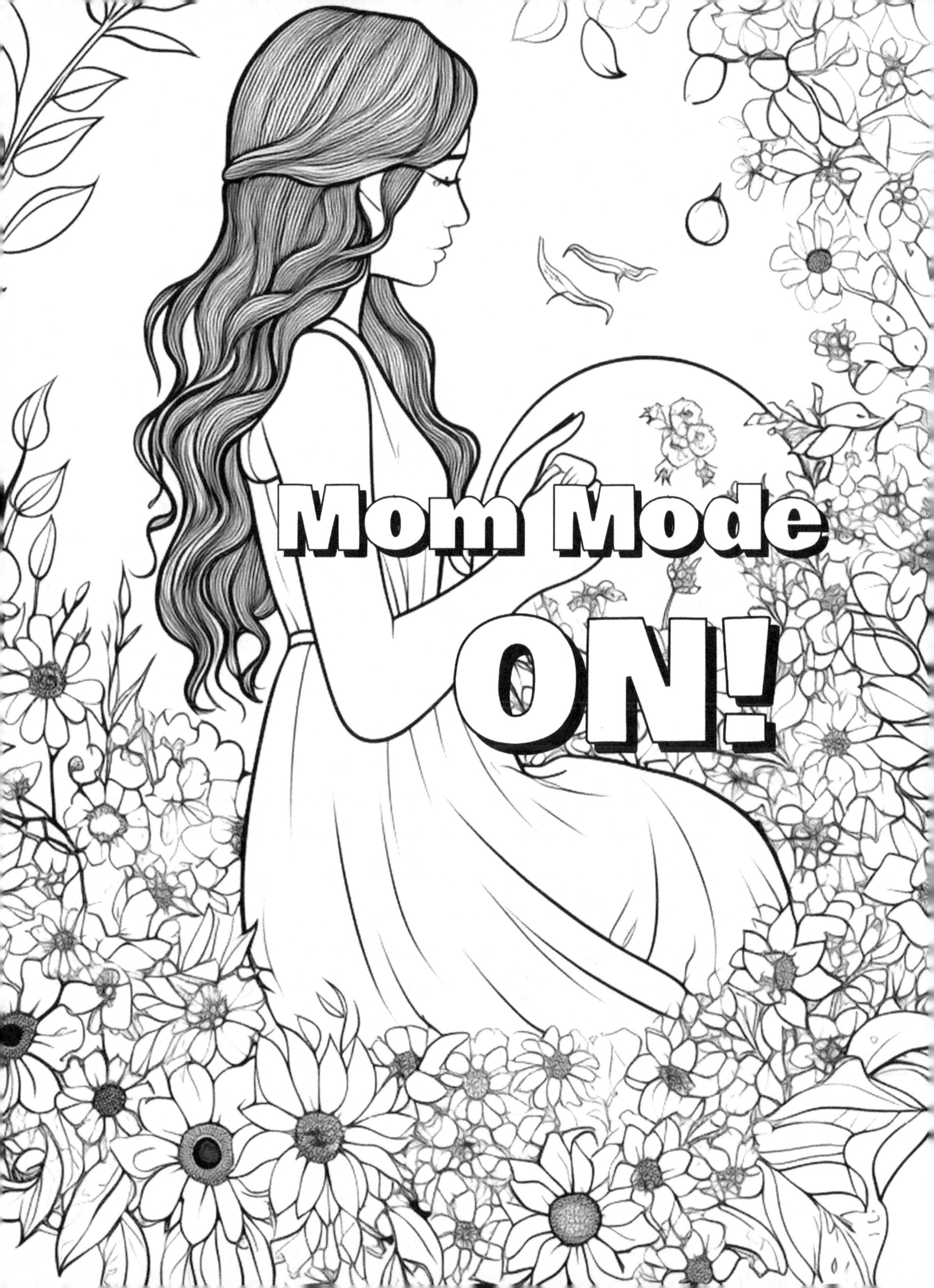

Mom Mode
ON!

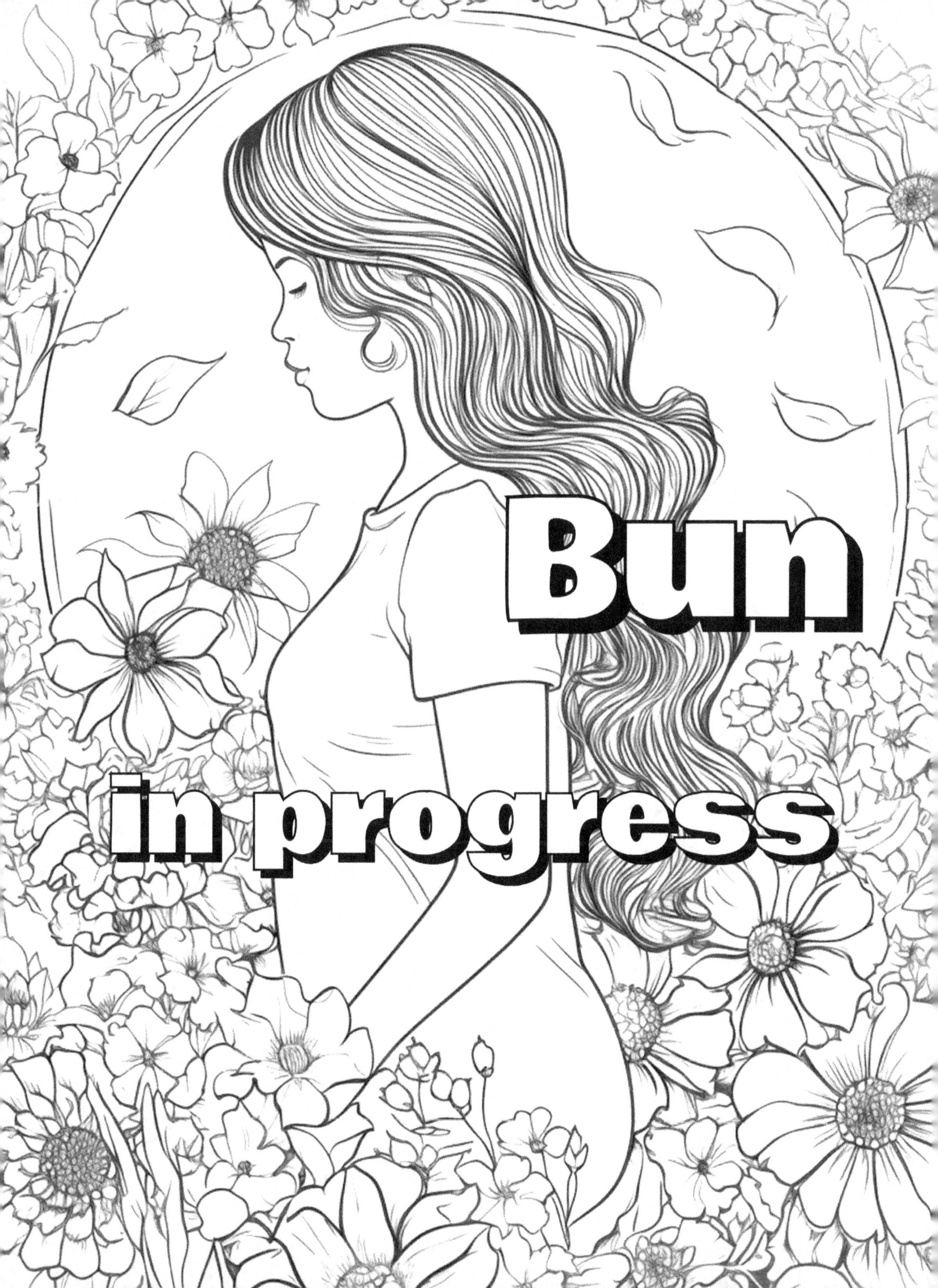

Bun
in progress

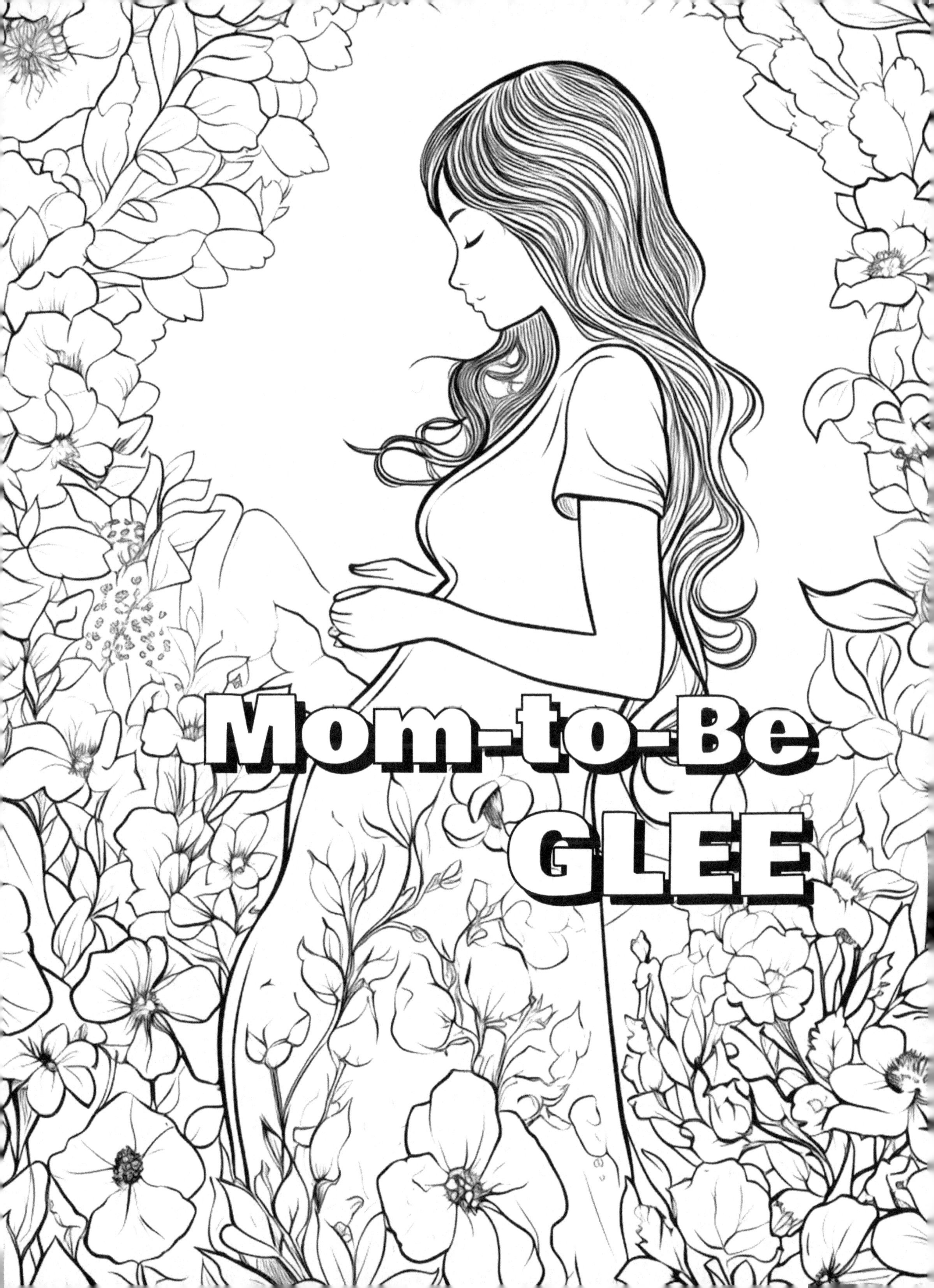
Mom-to-Be
GLEE

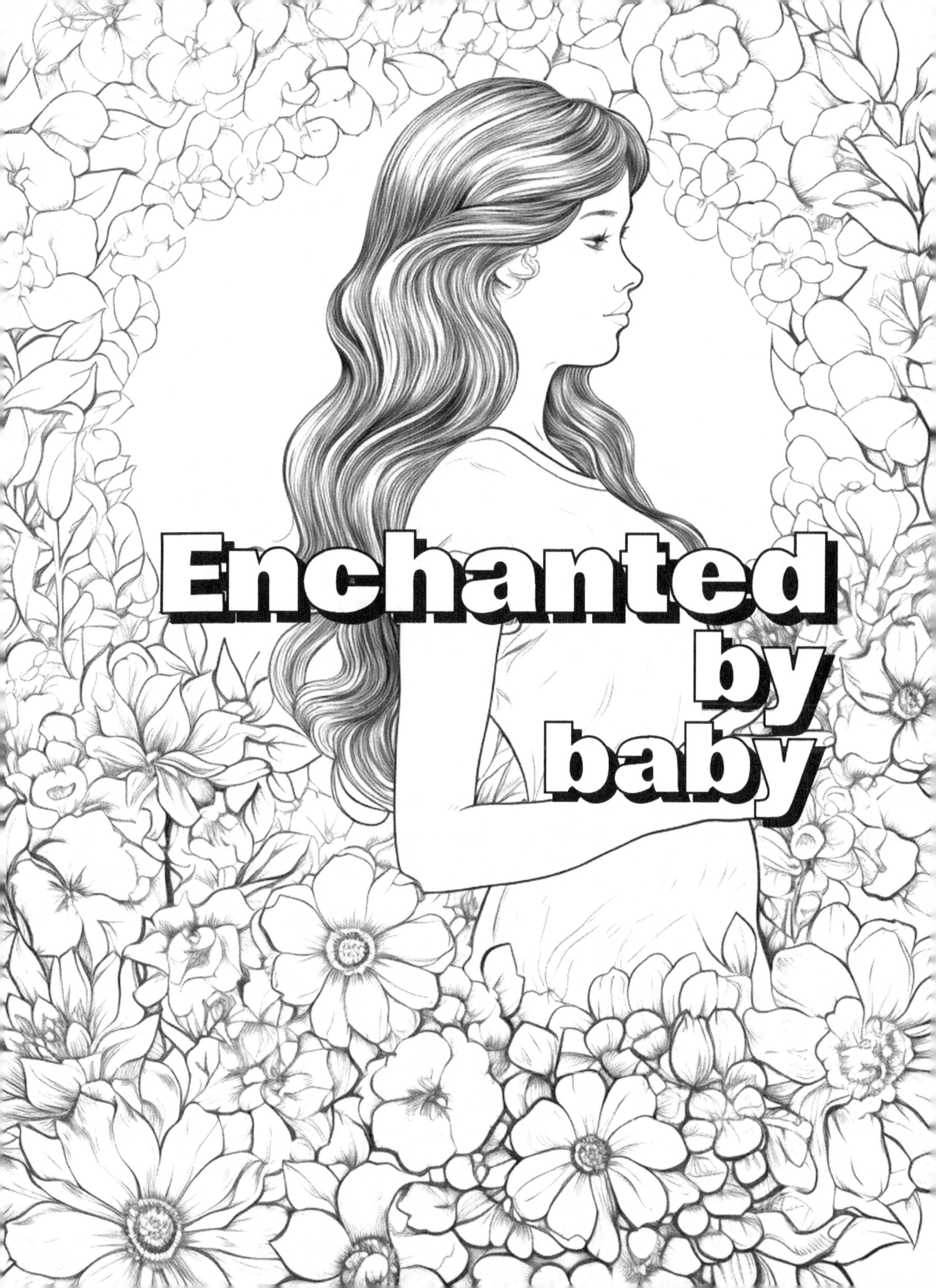
Enchanted
by
baby

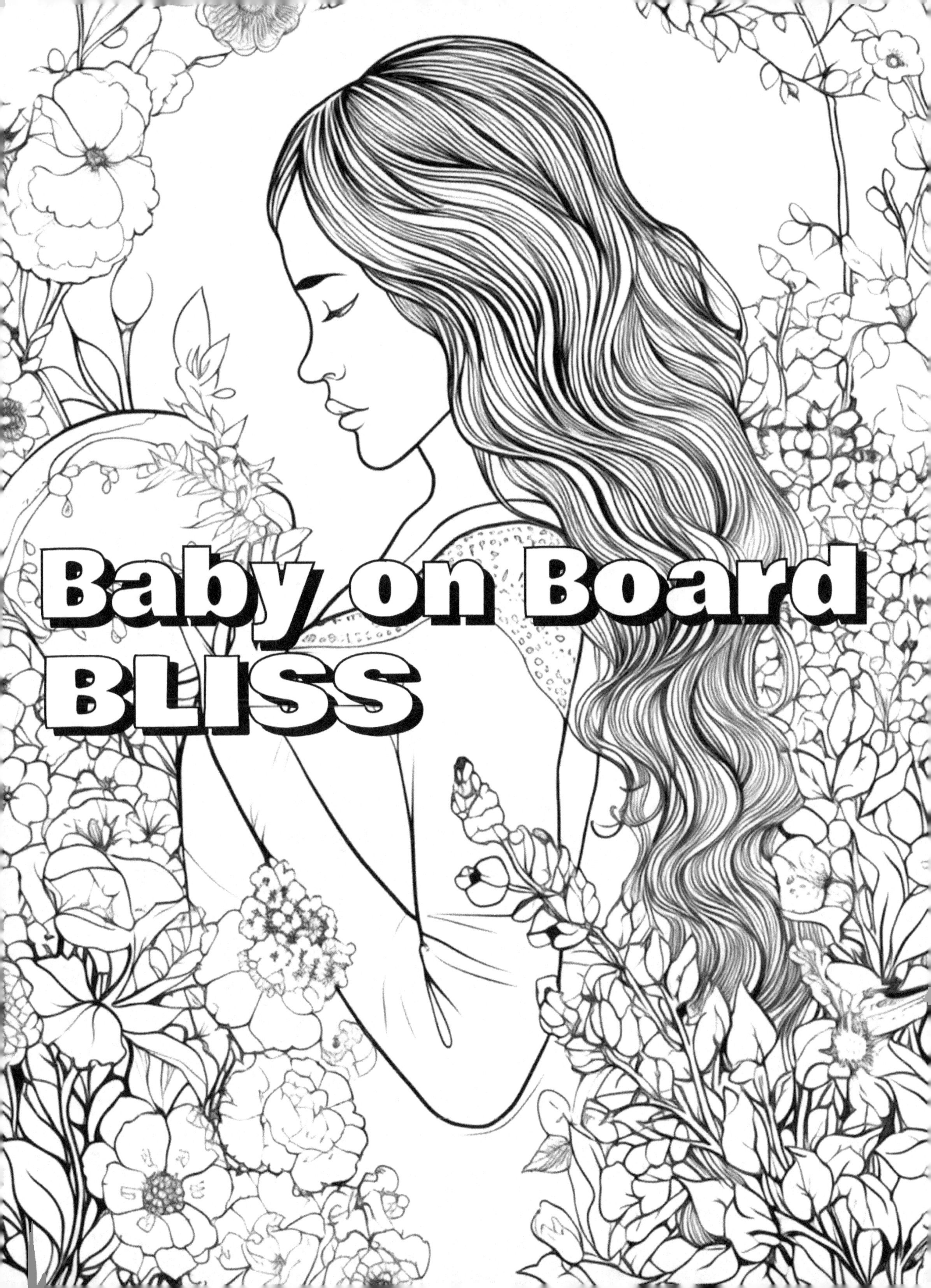

Baby on Board
BLISS

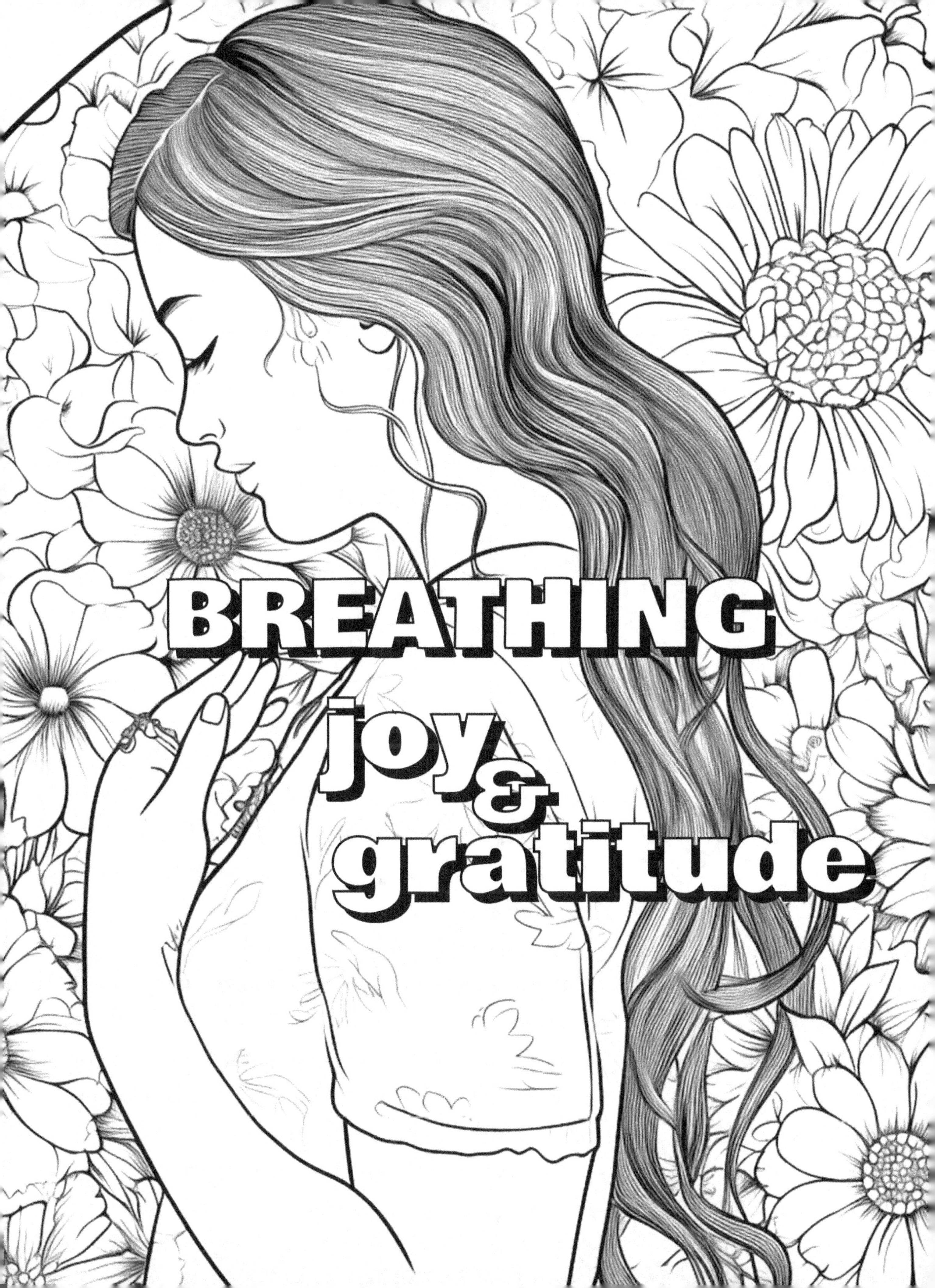
BREATHING
joy &
gratitude

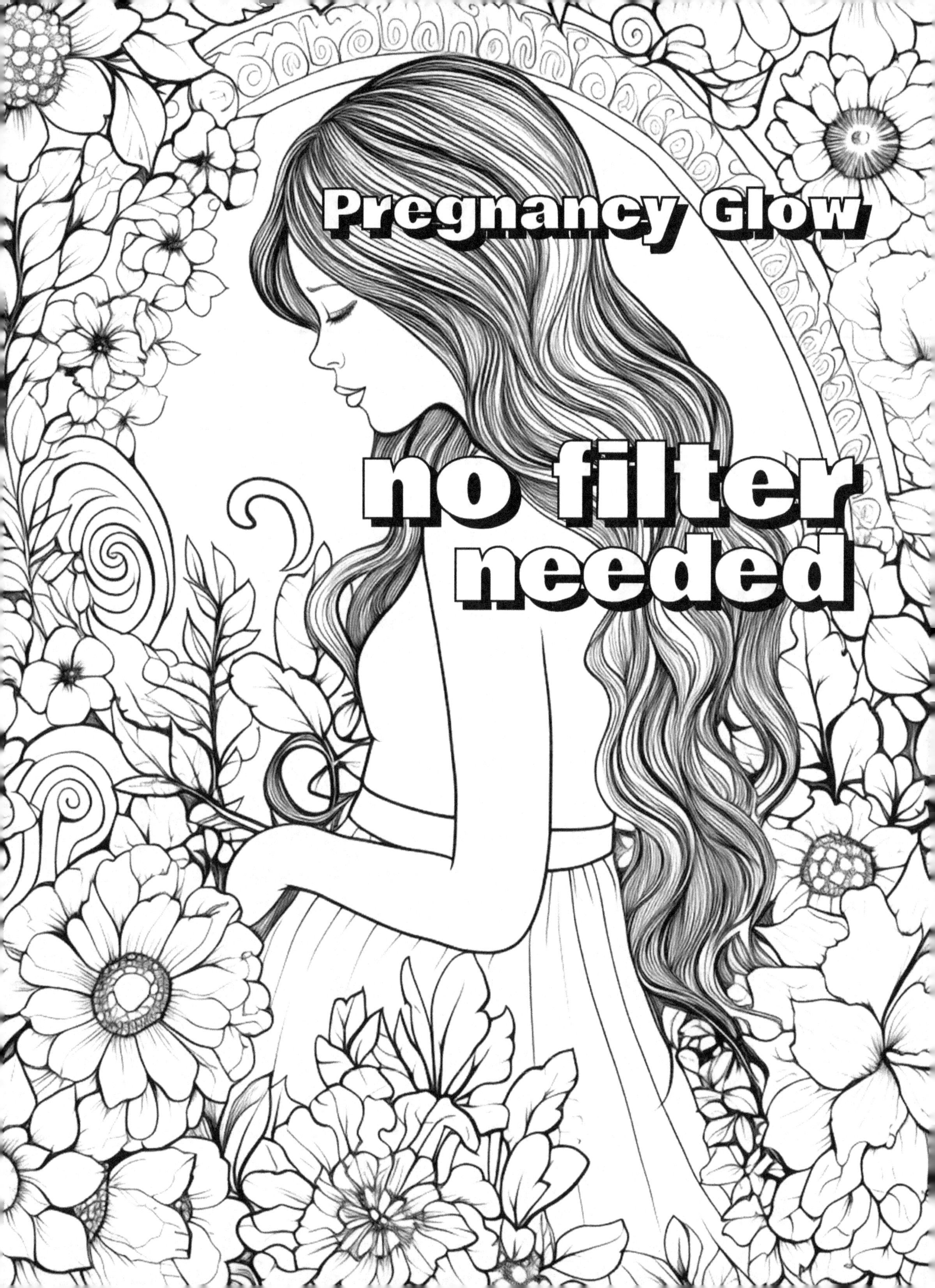

Pregnancy Glow
no filter
needed

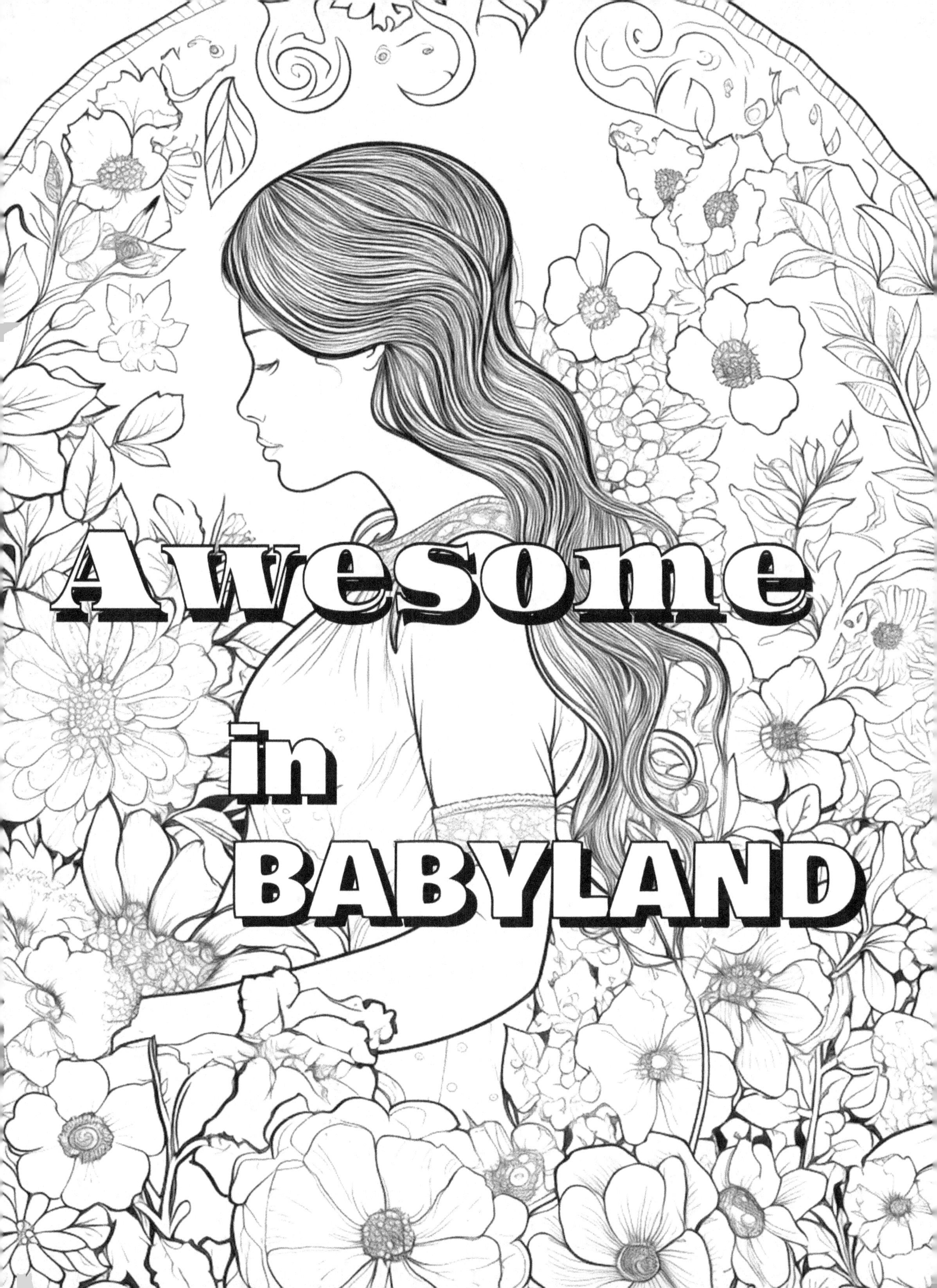

Awesome
in
BABYLAND

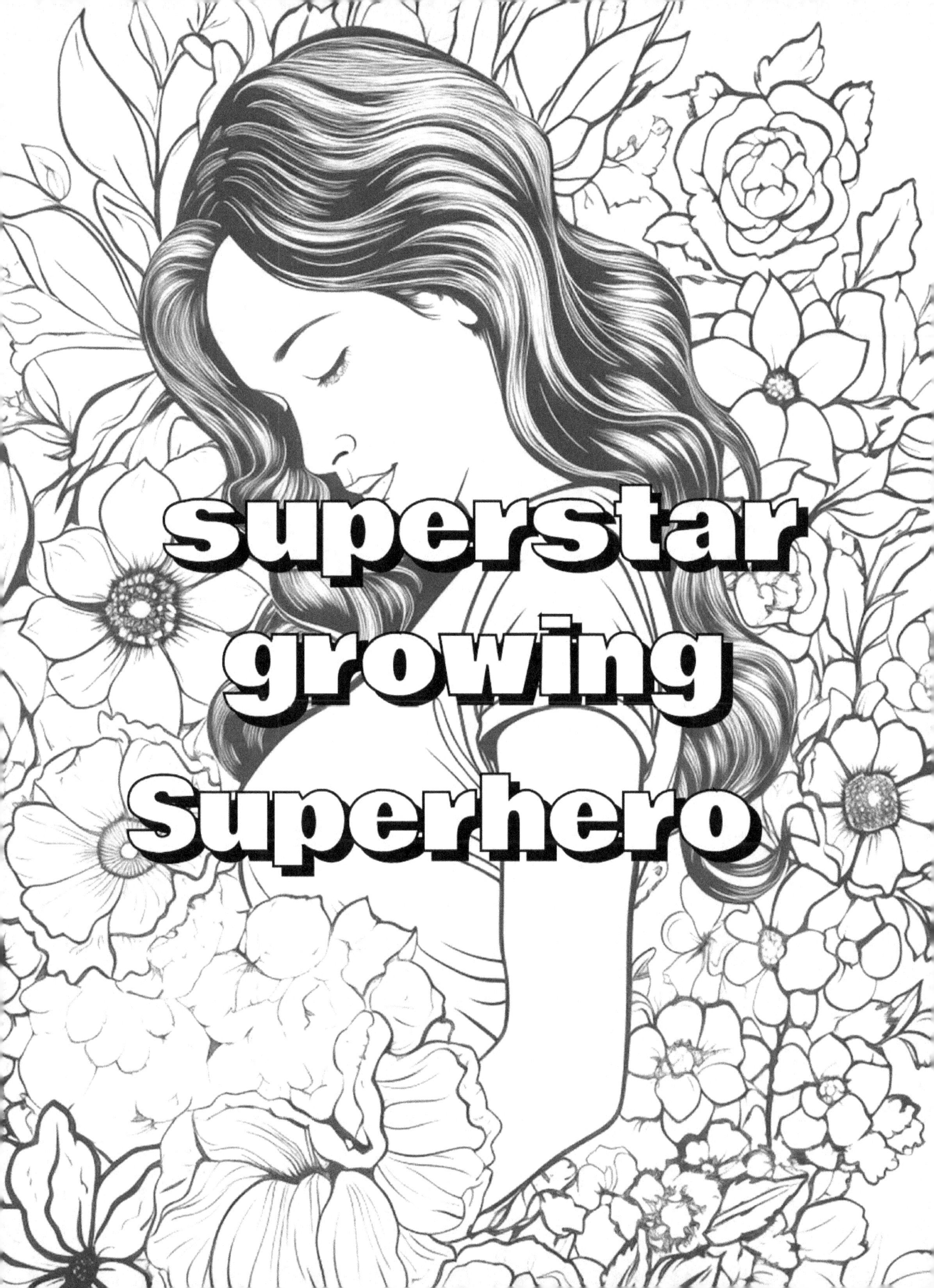

superstar
growing
Superhero

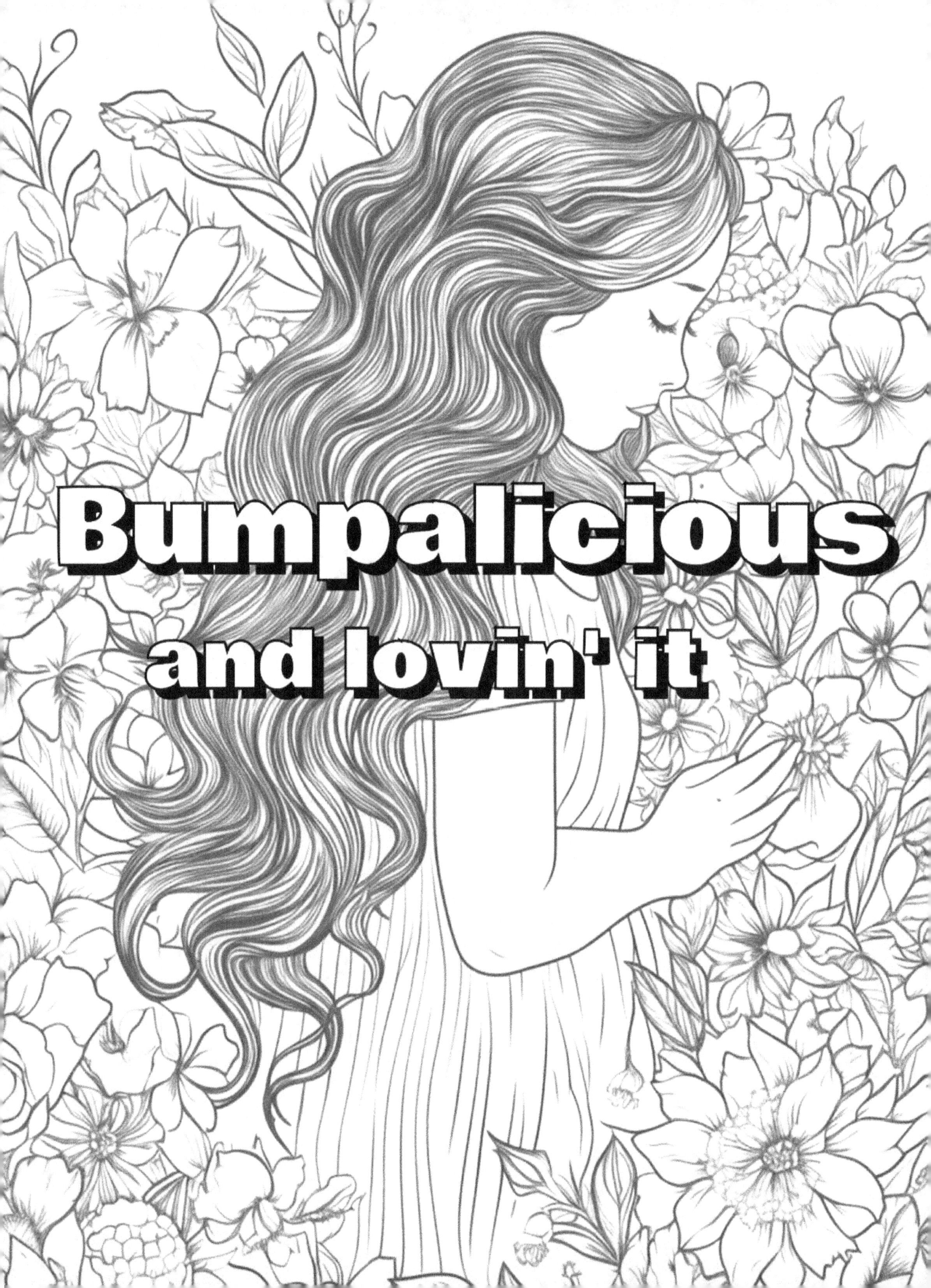
Bumpalicious
and lovin' it

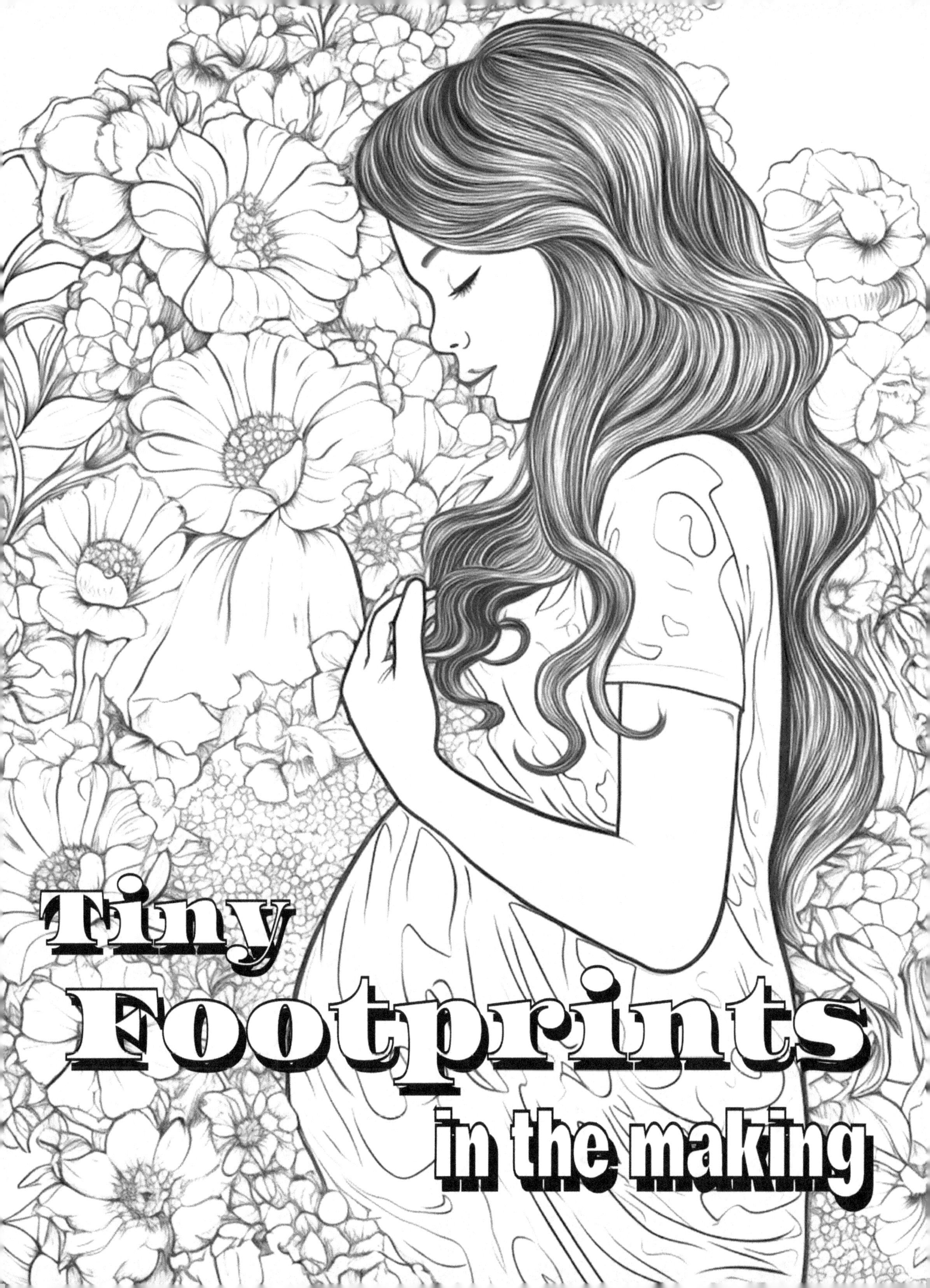

Tiny
Footprints
in the making

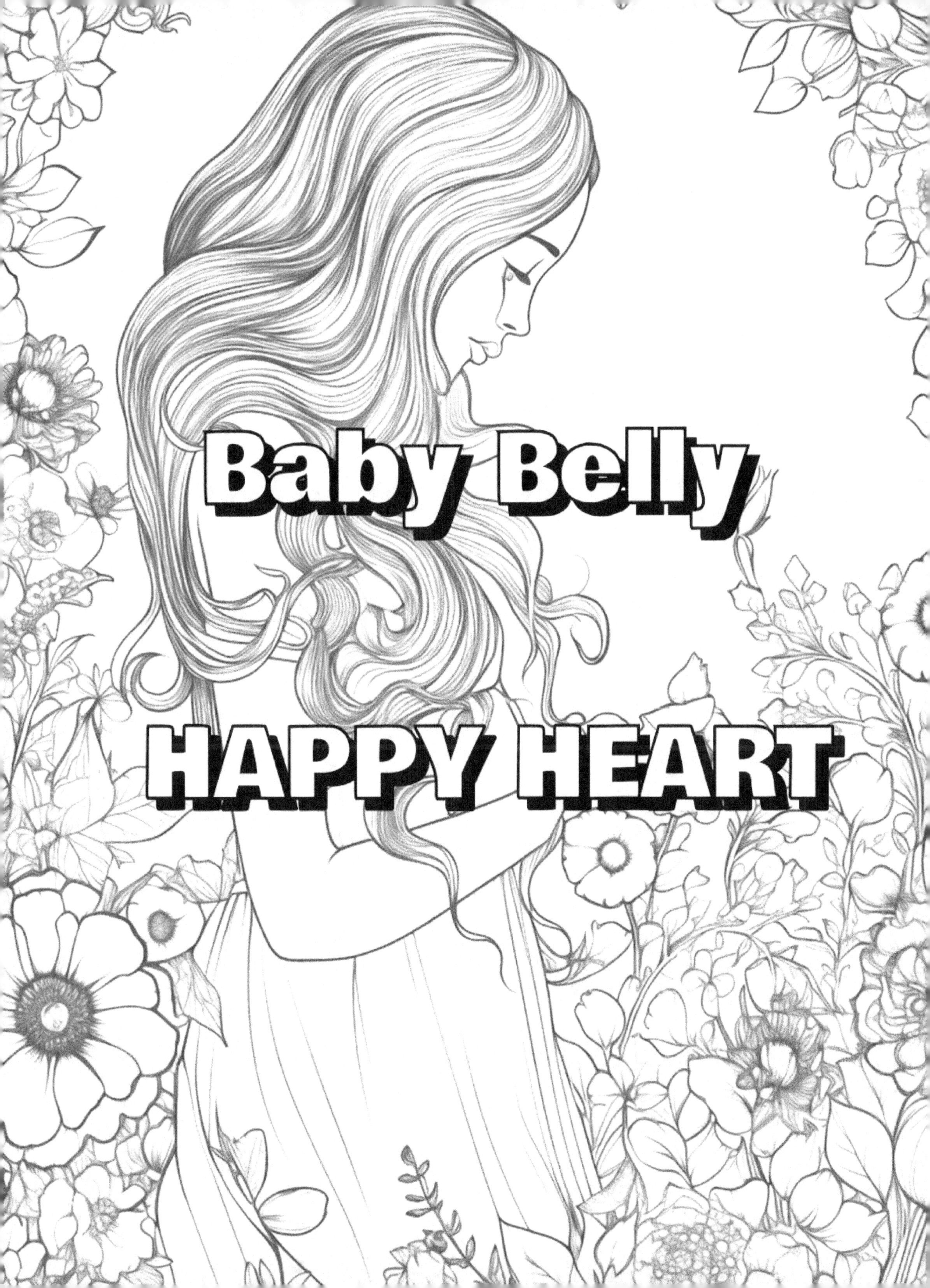
Baby Belly
HAPPY HEART

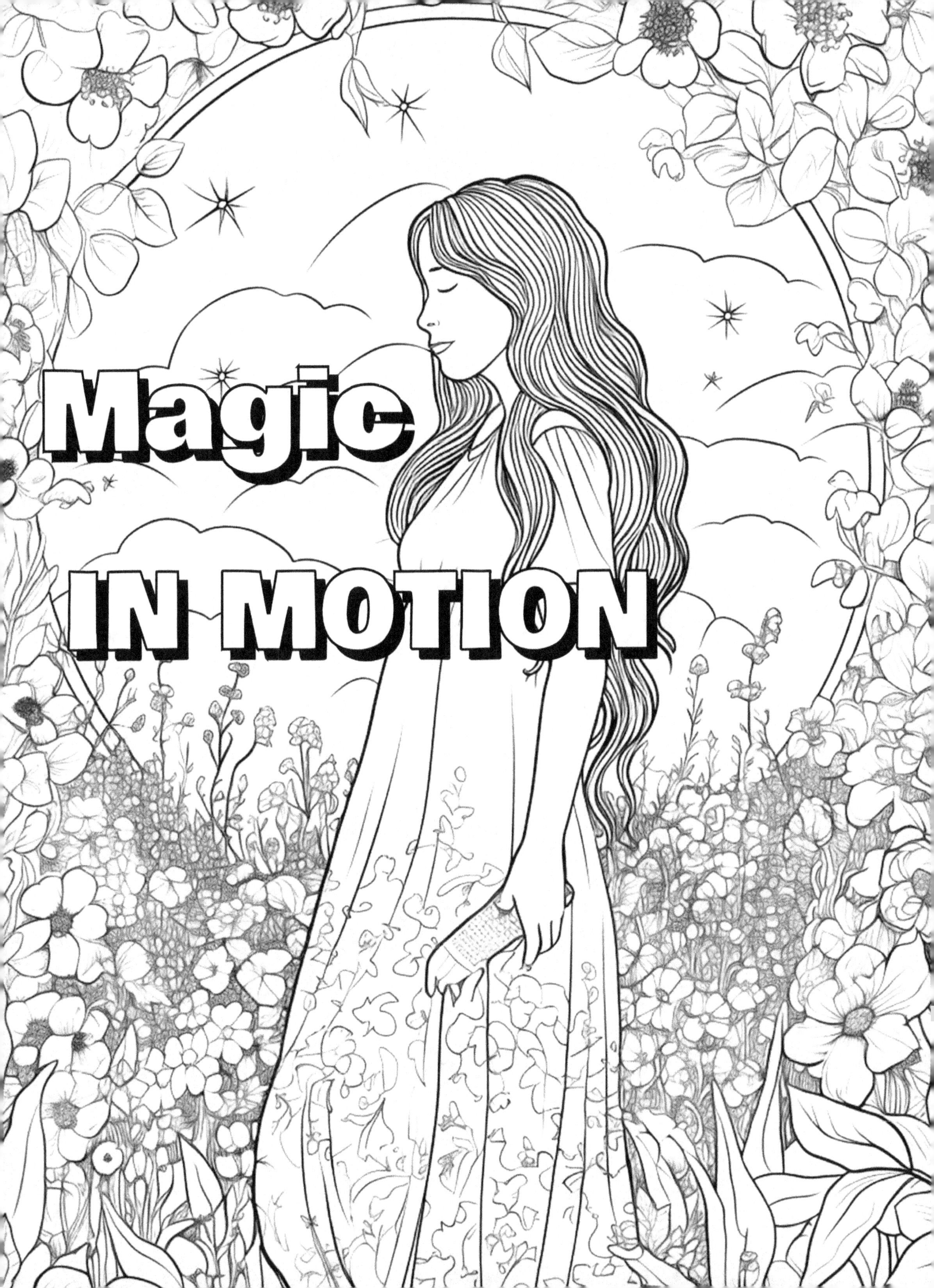

Magic
IN MOTION

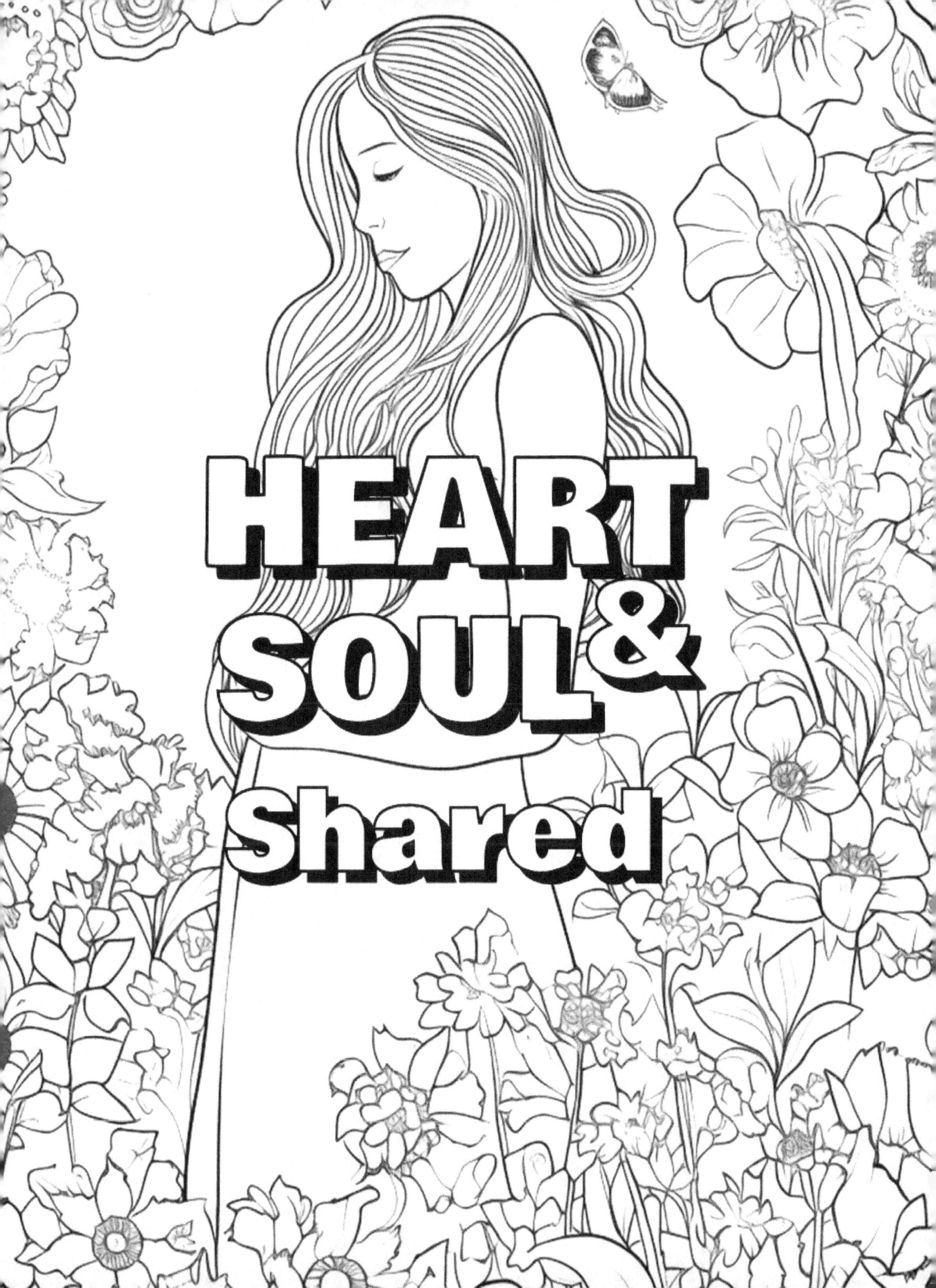

HEART
SOUL &
Shared

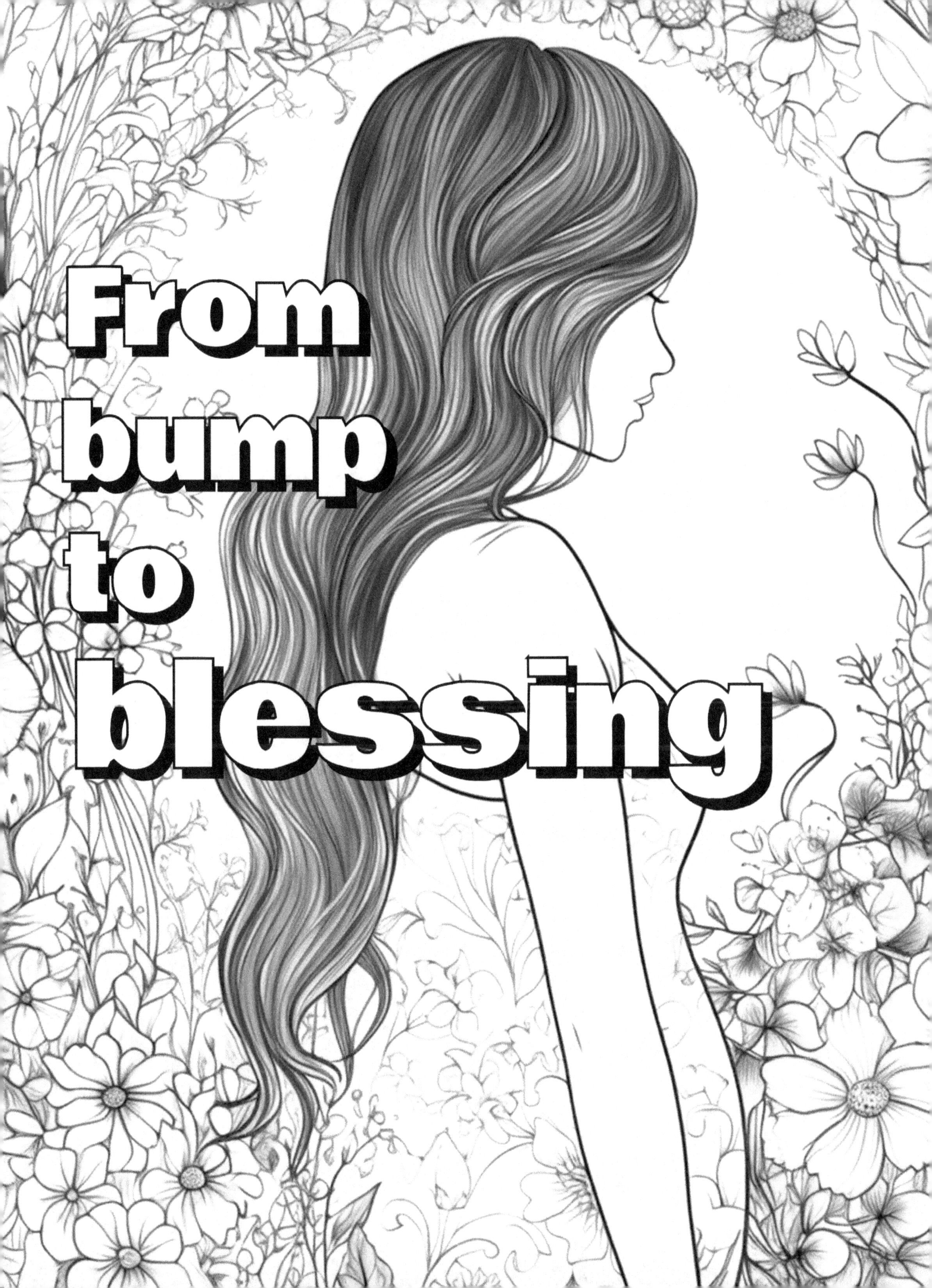

From
bump
to
blessing

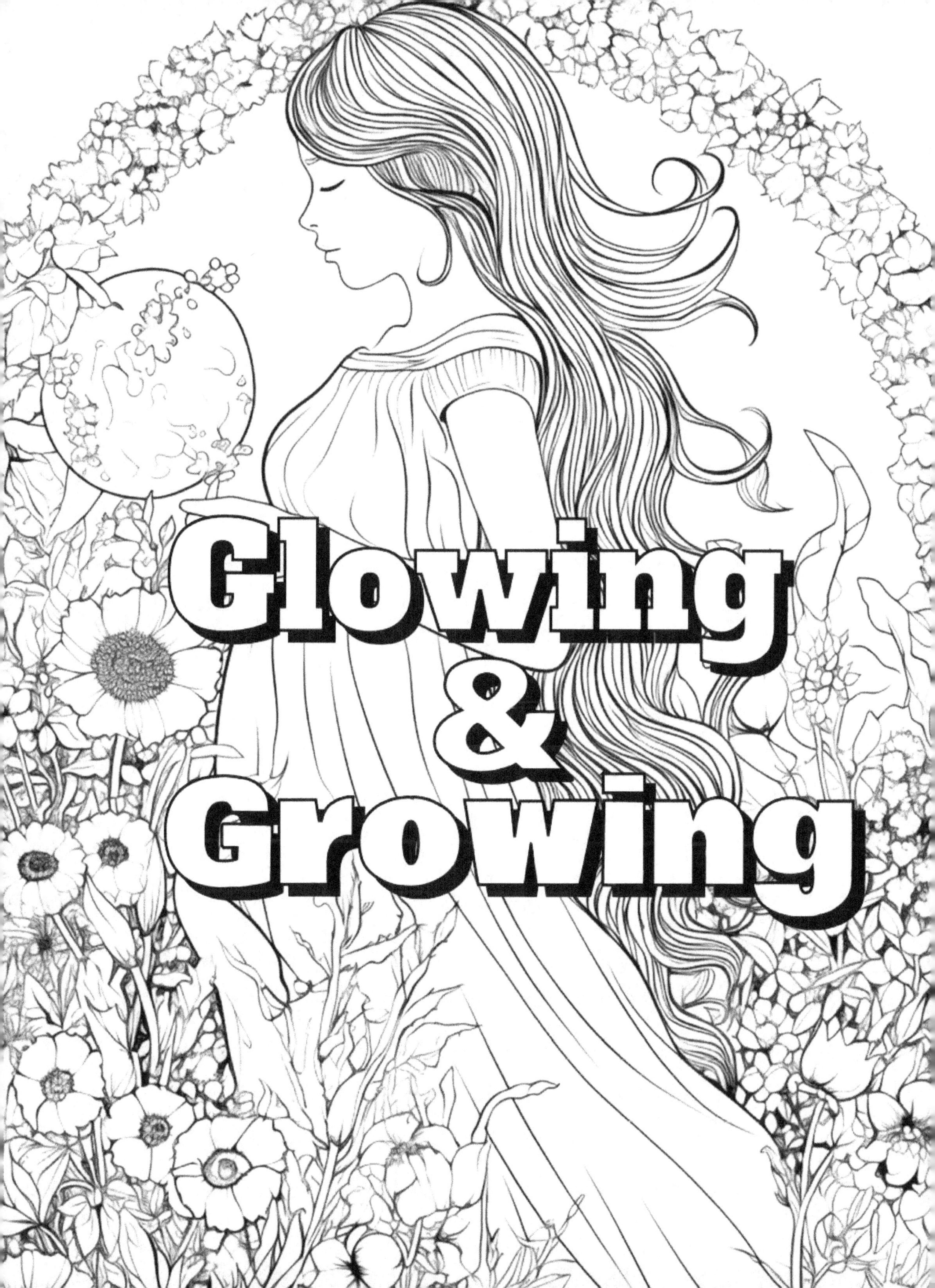
Glowing
&
Growing

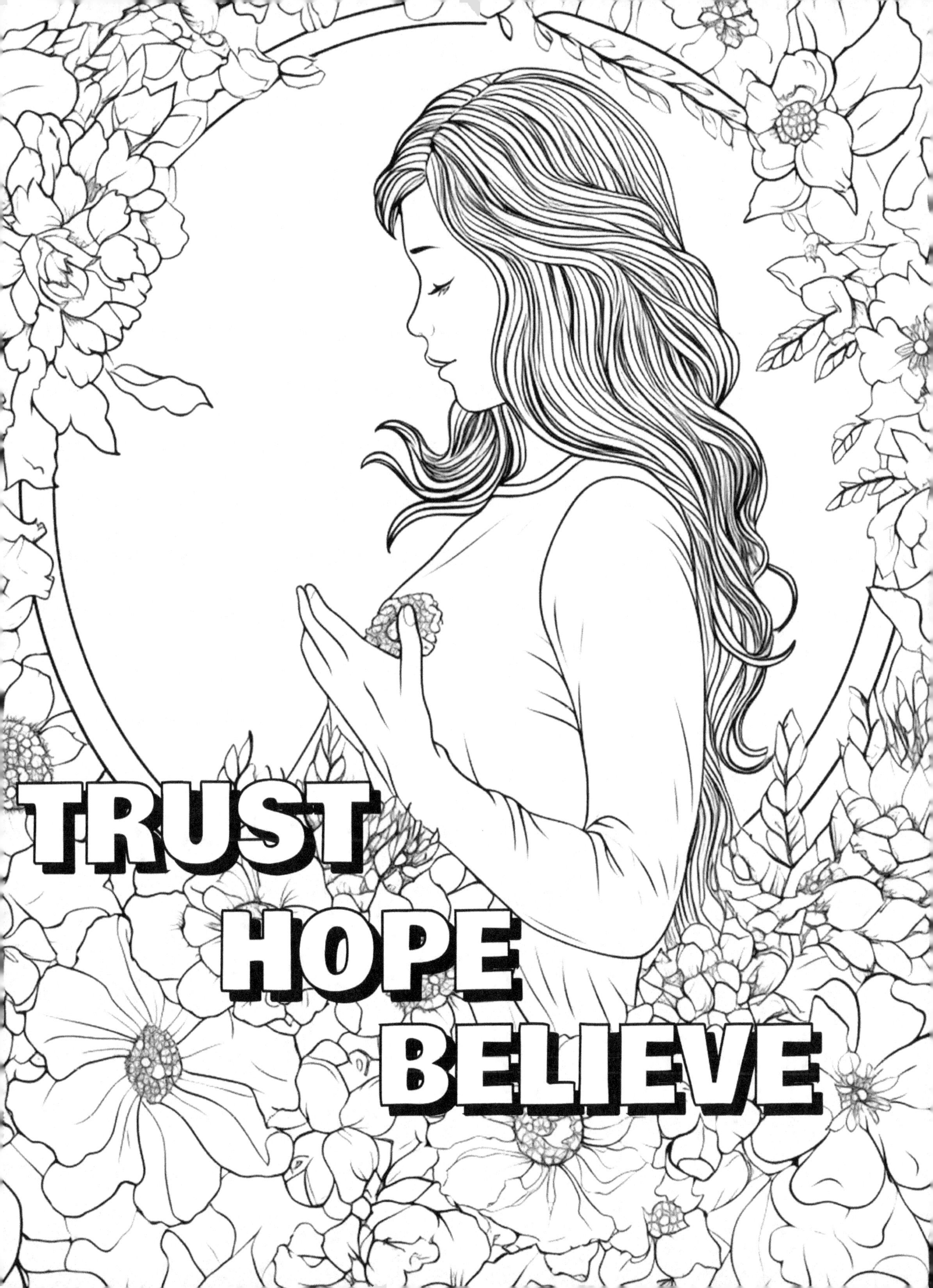

TRUST
HOPE
BELIEVE

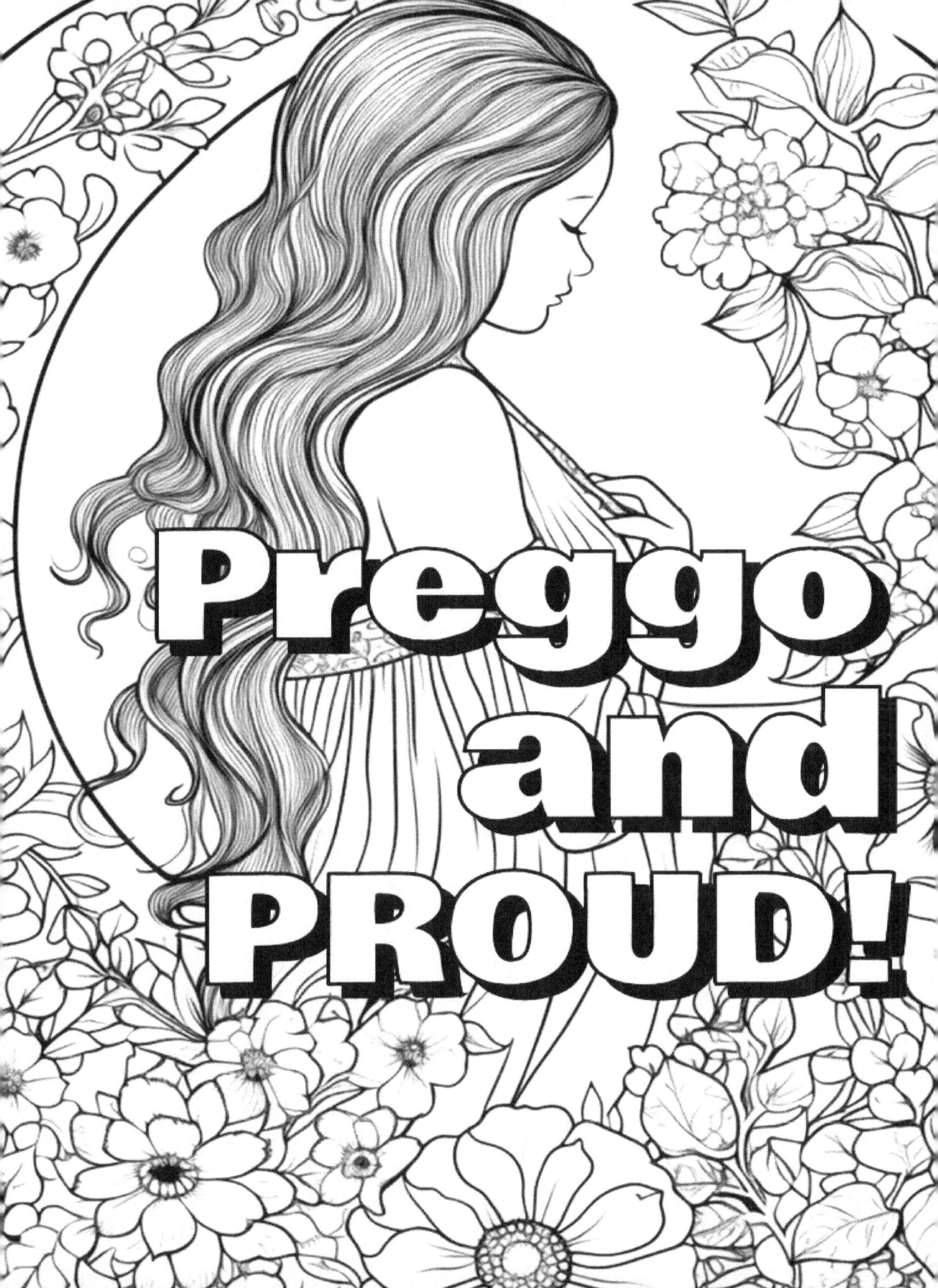

Preggo
and
PROUD!

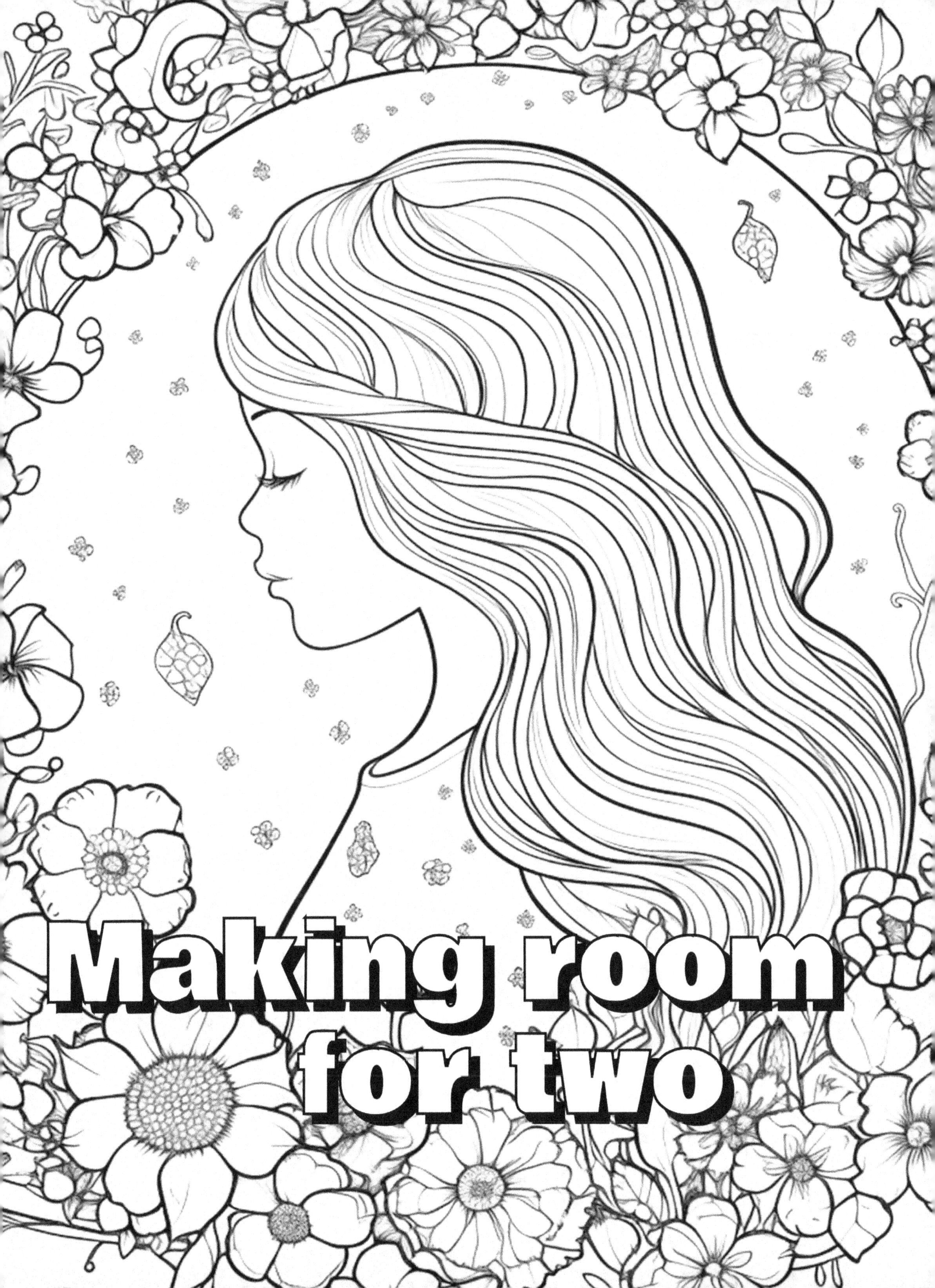
Making room
for two

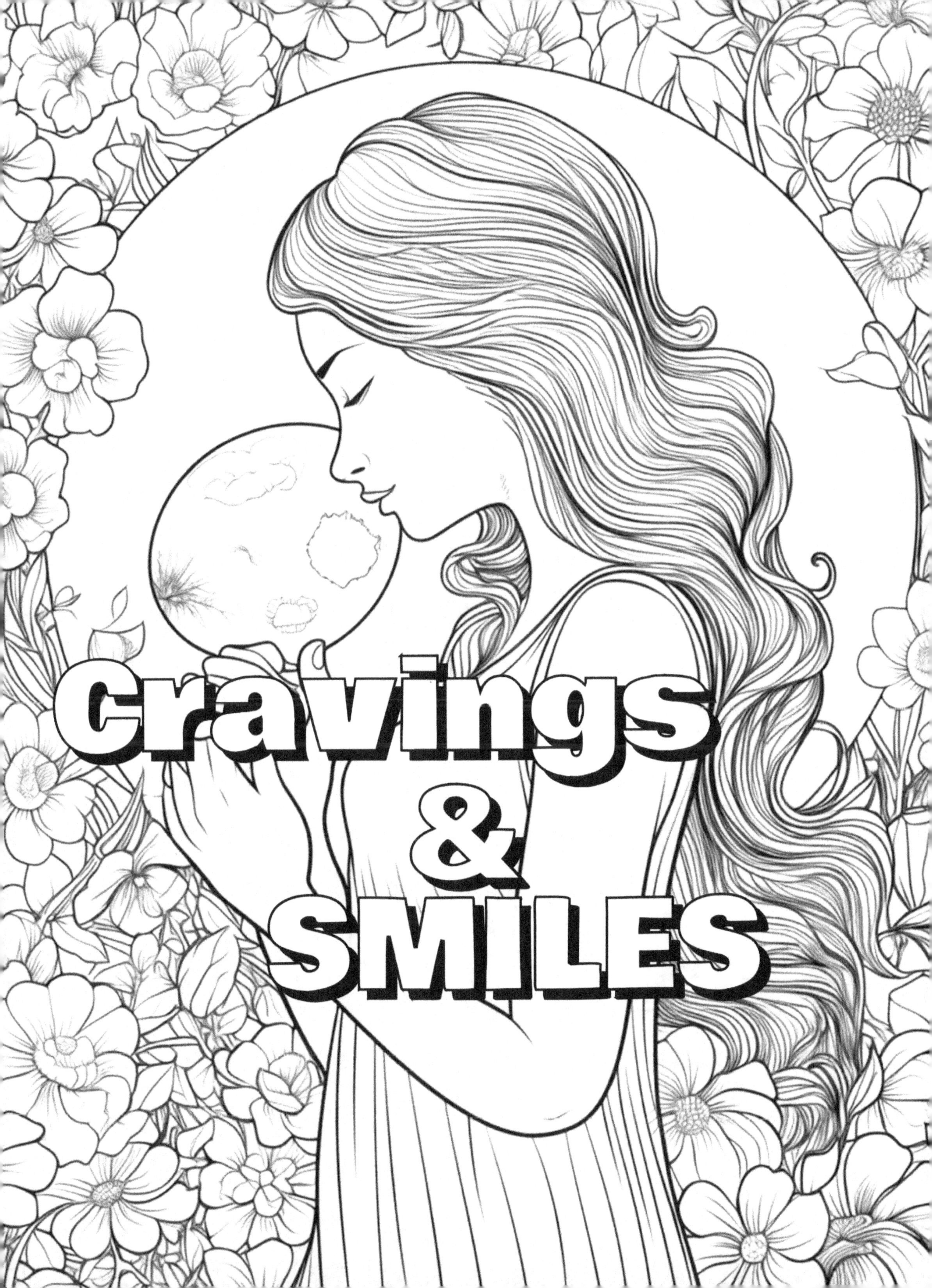

Cravings
&
SMILES

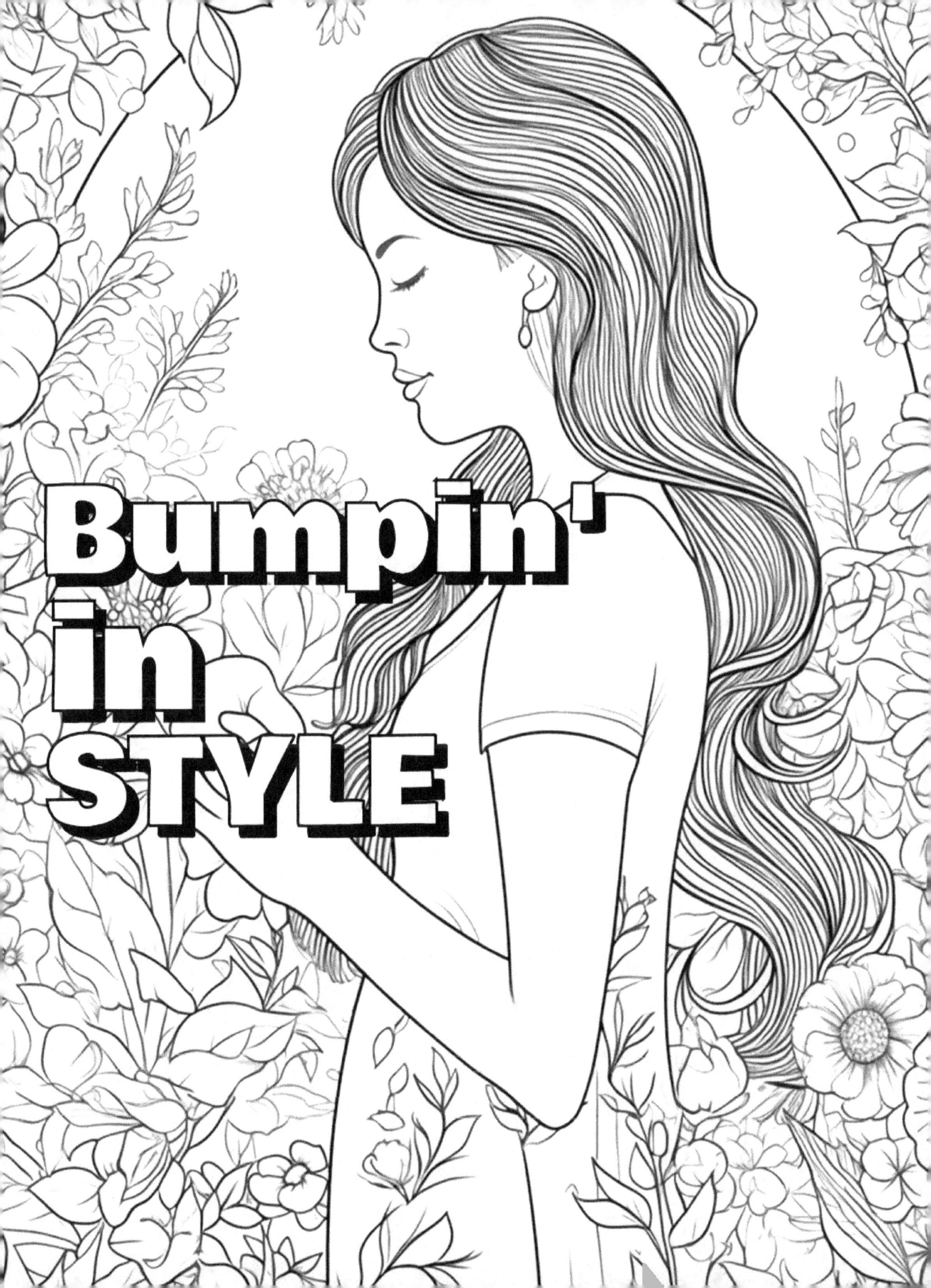

Bumpin'
in
STYLE

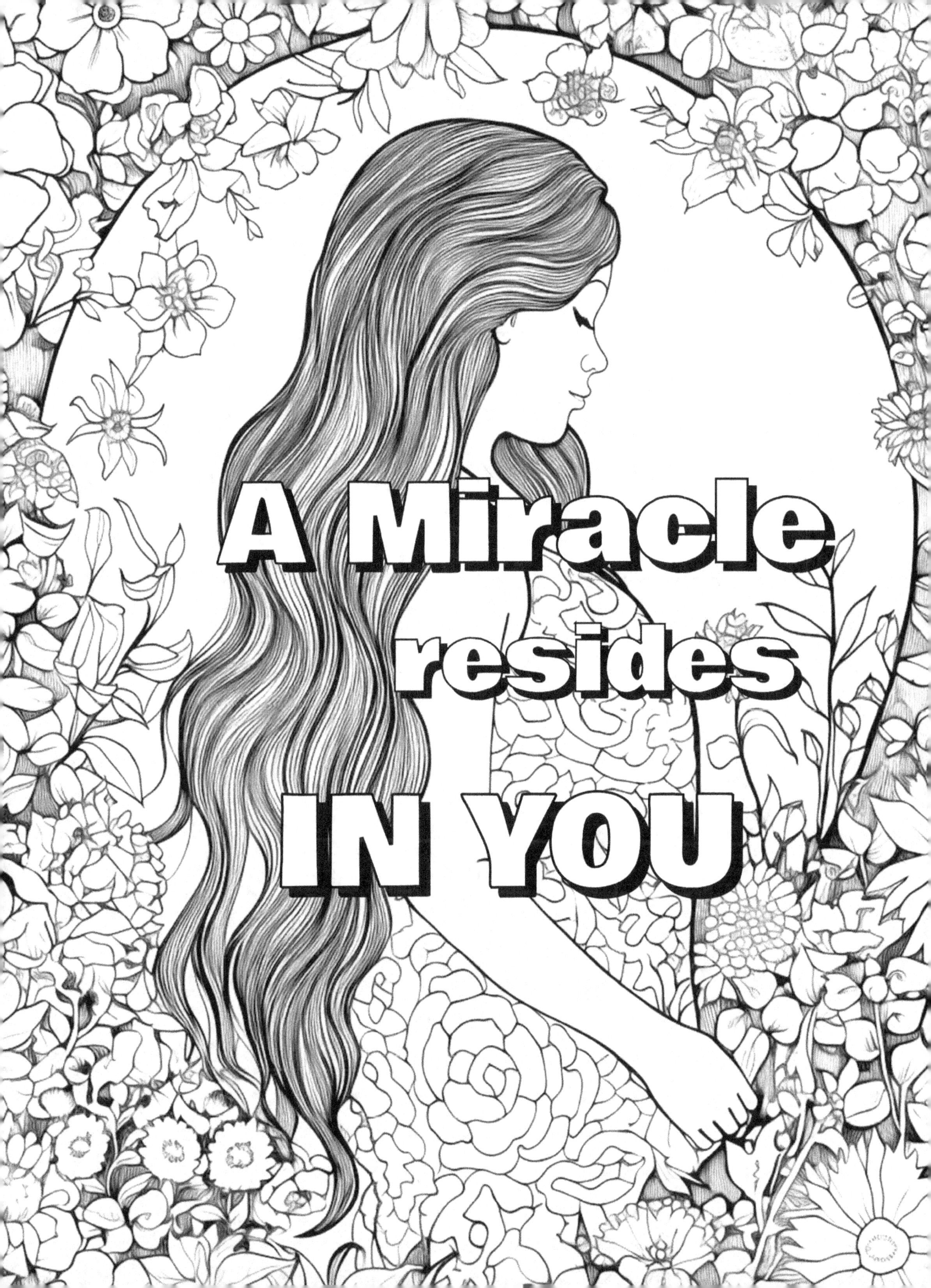

A Miracle
resides
IN YOU

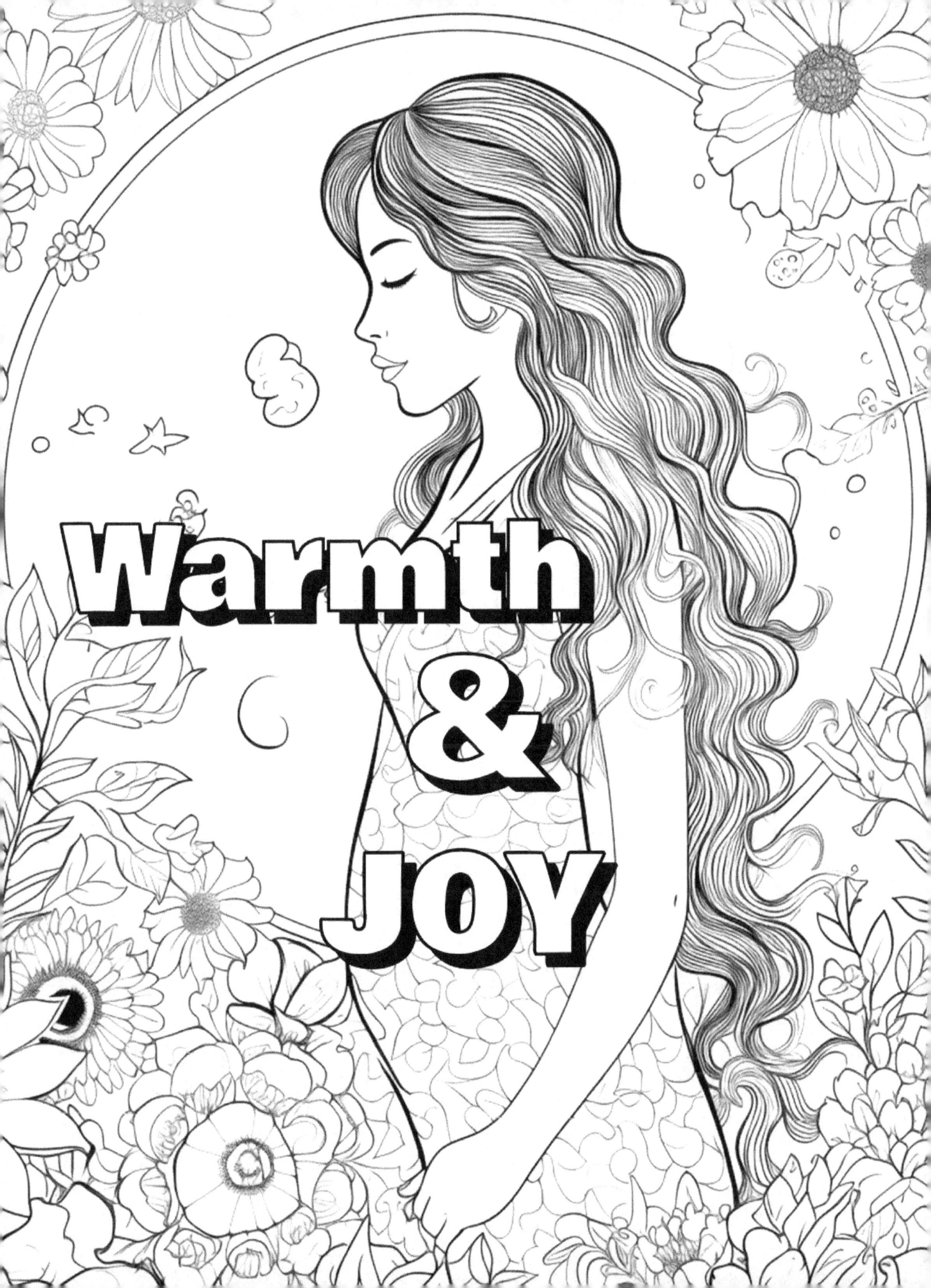

Warmth
&
JOY

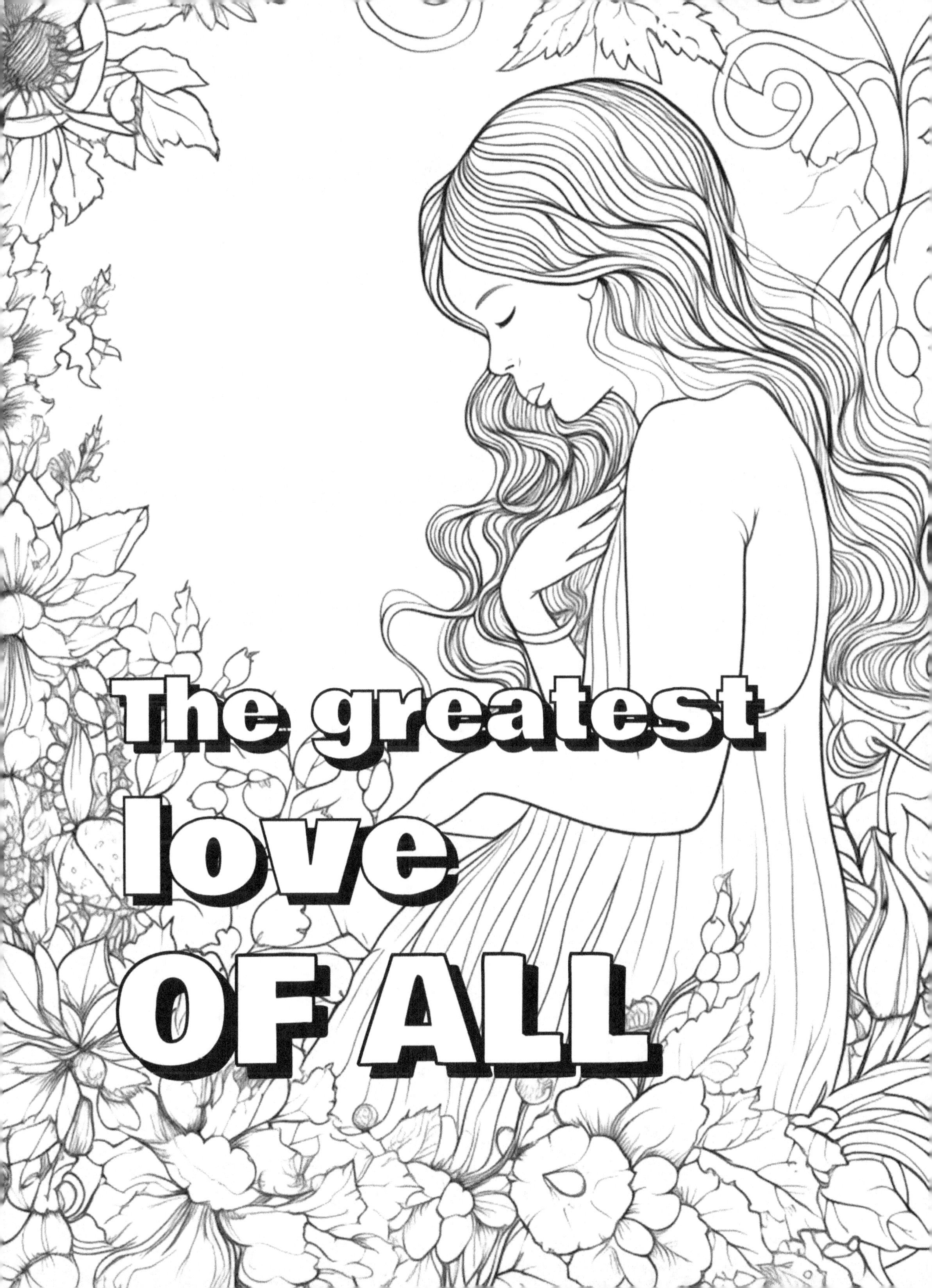

The greatest
love
OF ALL

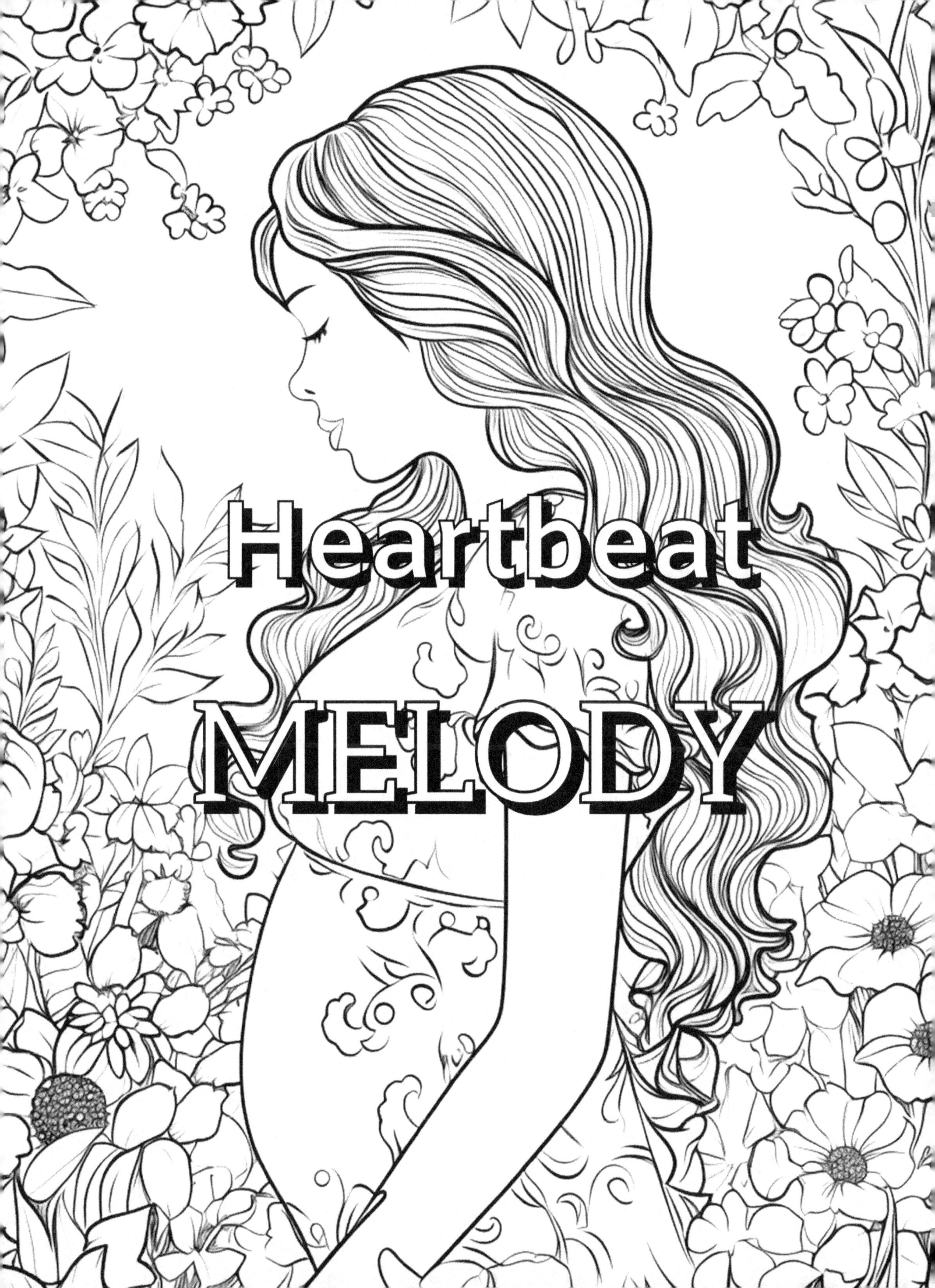

Heartbeat
MELODY

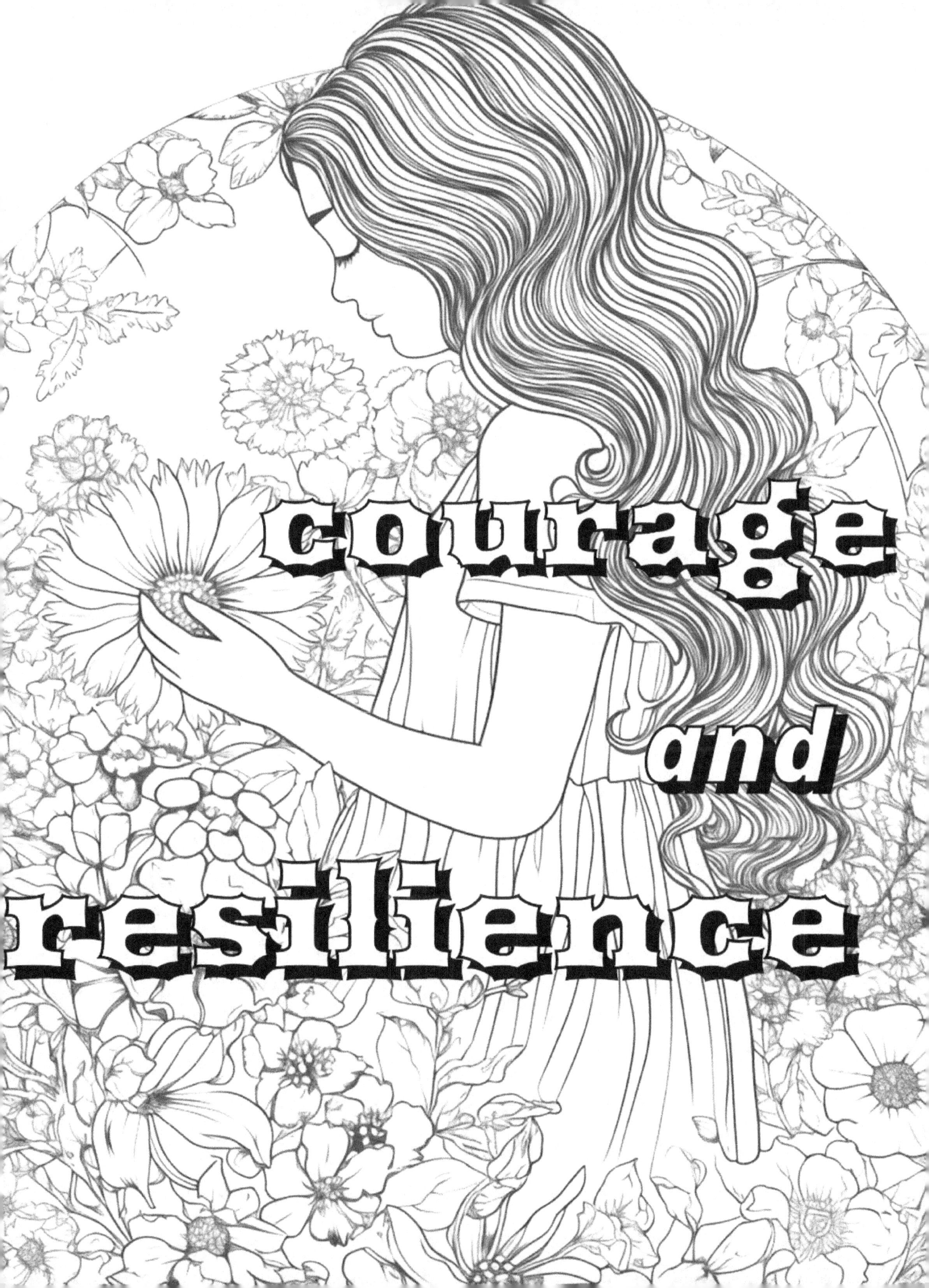
courage
and
resilience

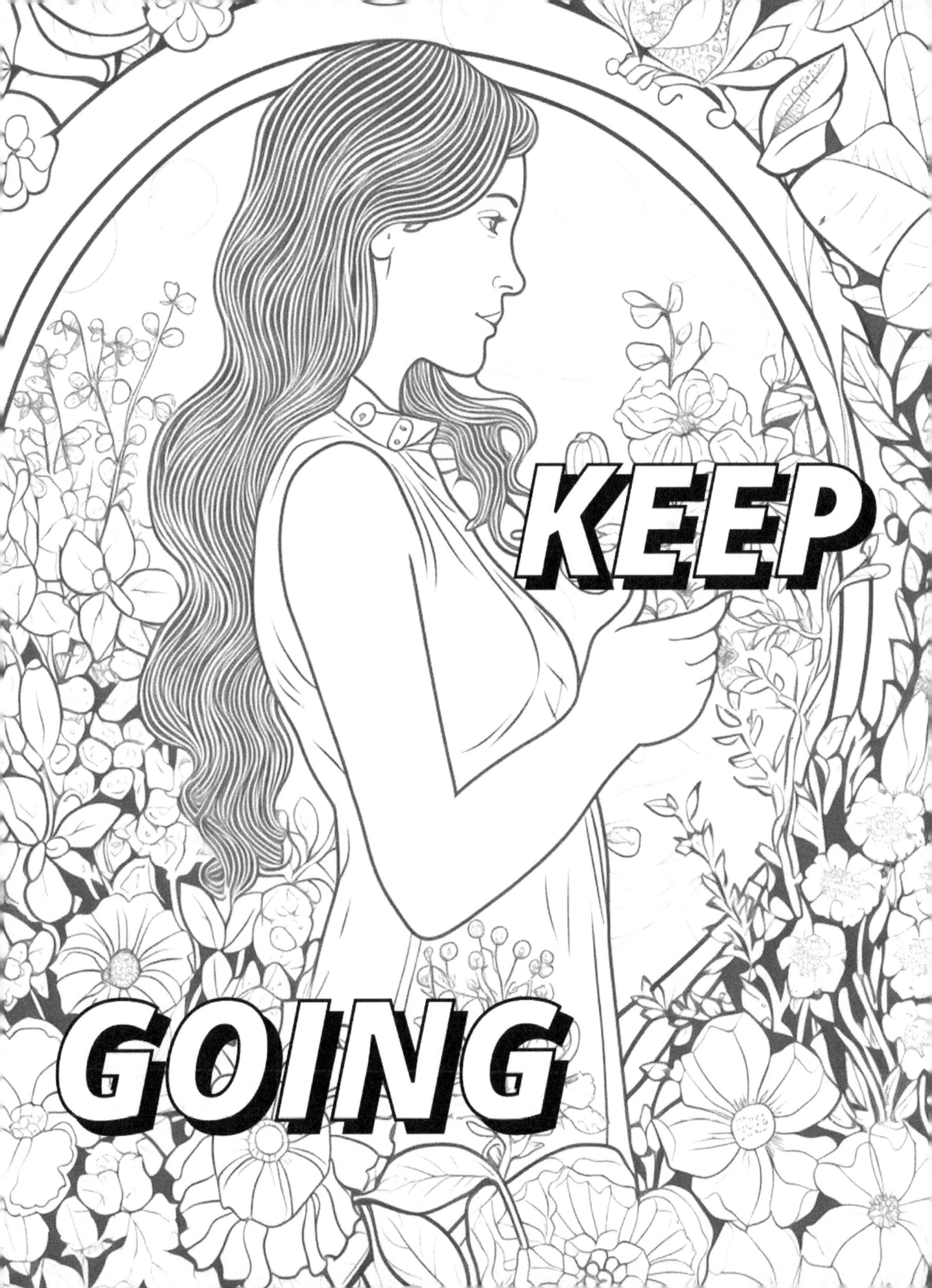

KEEP
GOING

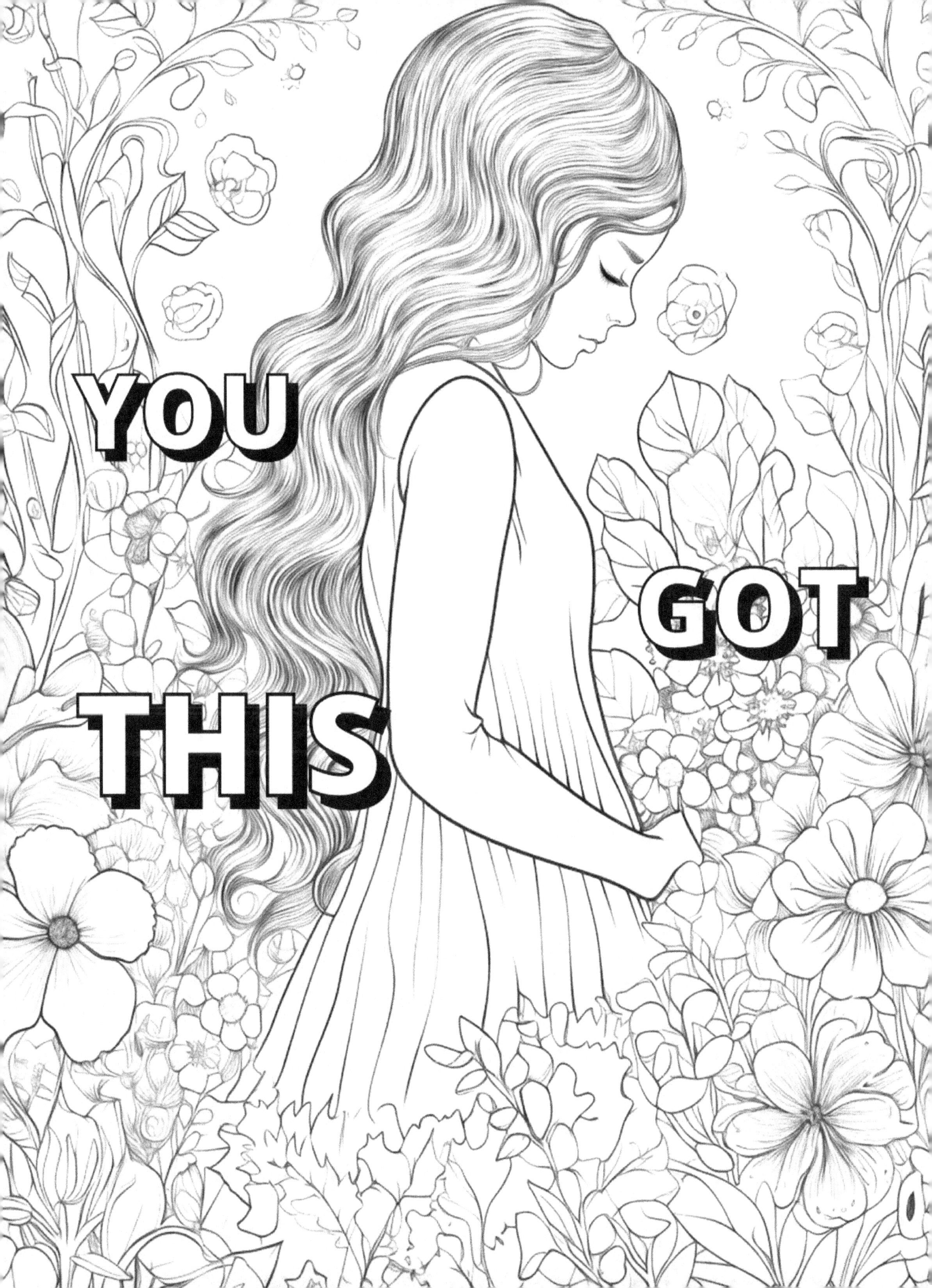

YOU
GOT
THIS

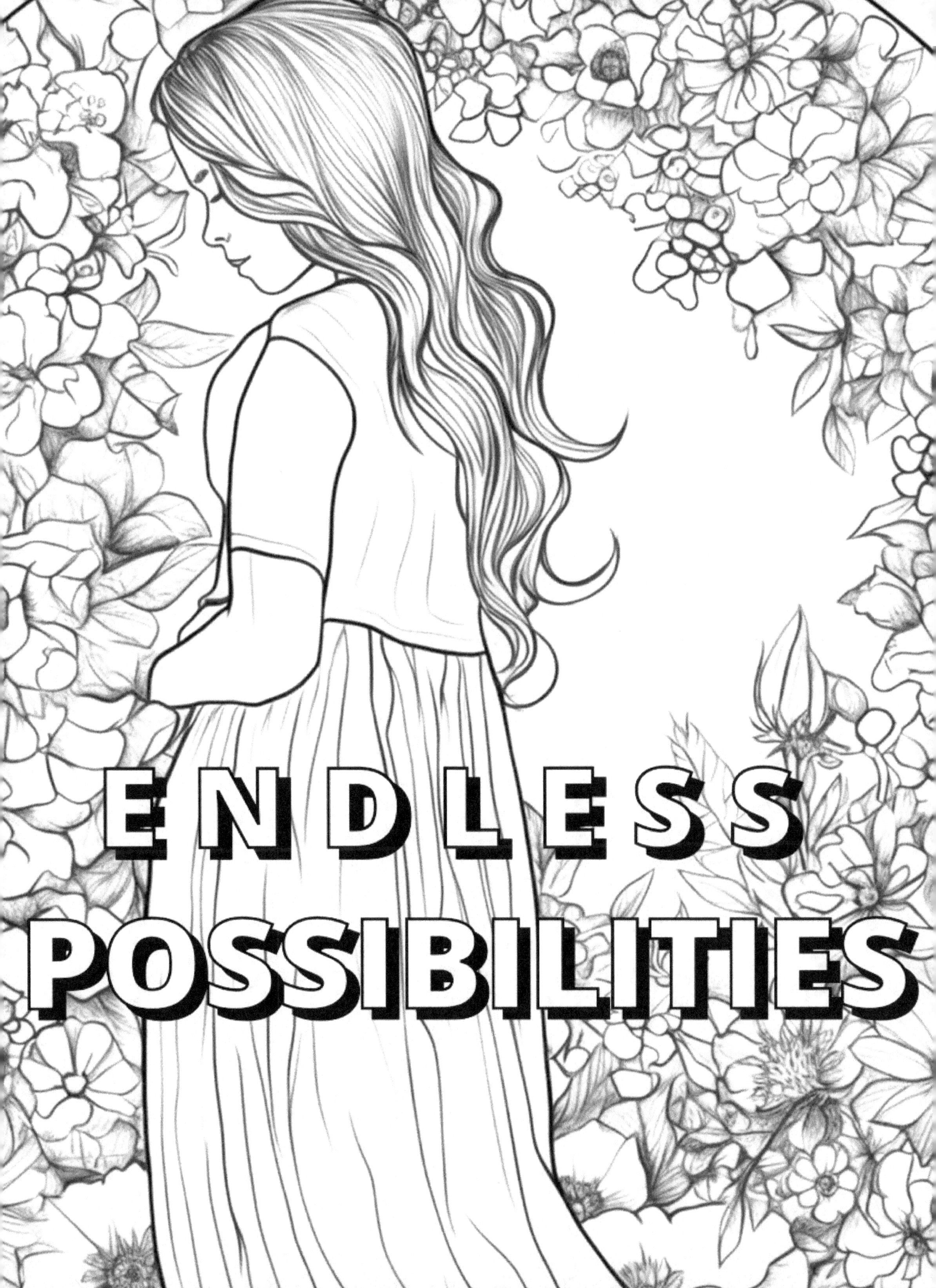
ENDLESS
POSSIBILITIES

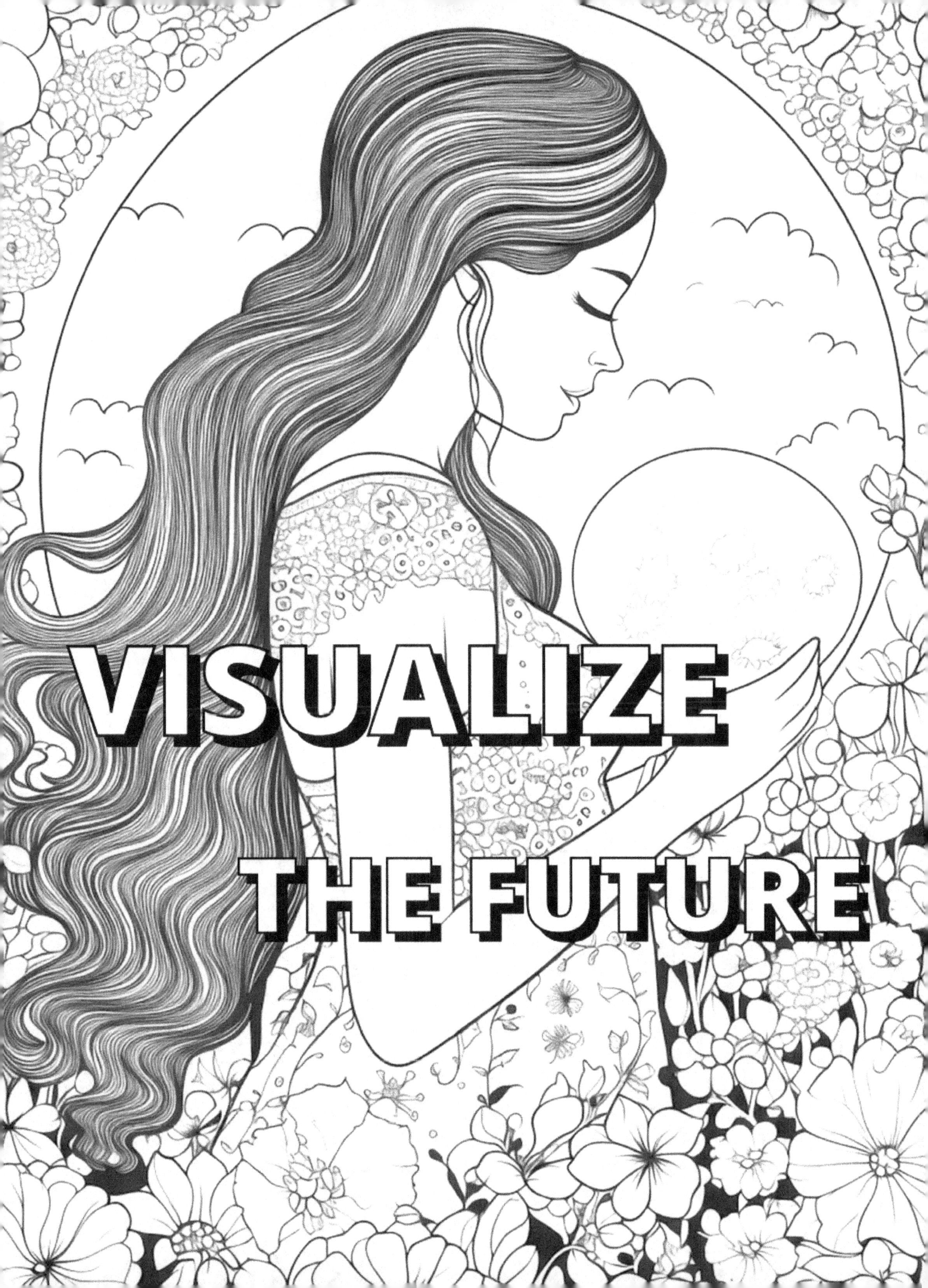

VISUALIZE
THE FUTURE

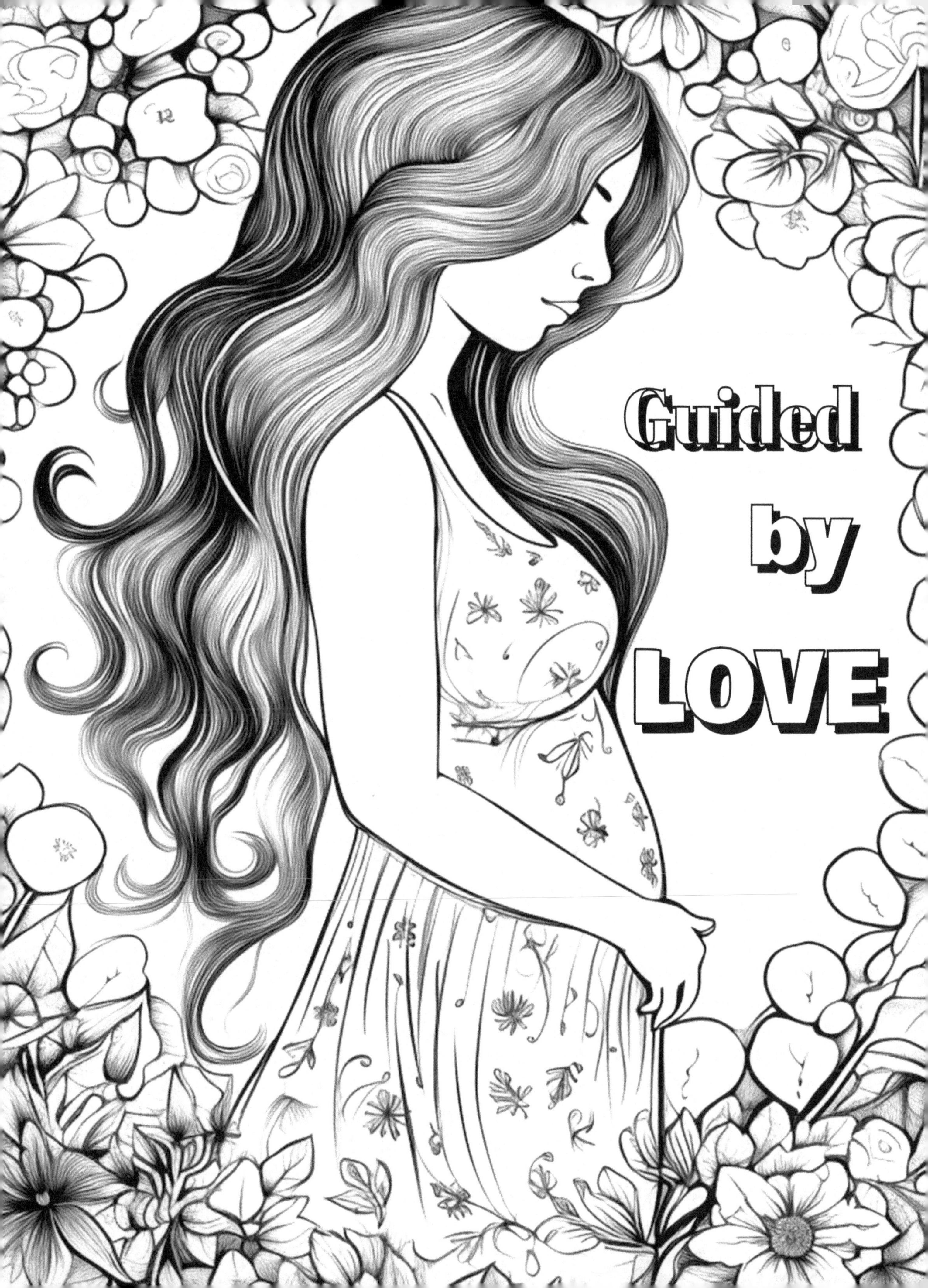

Guided
by
LOVE

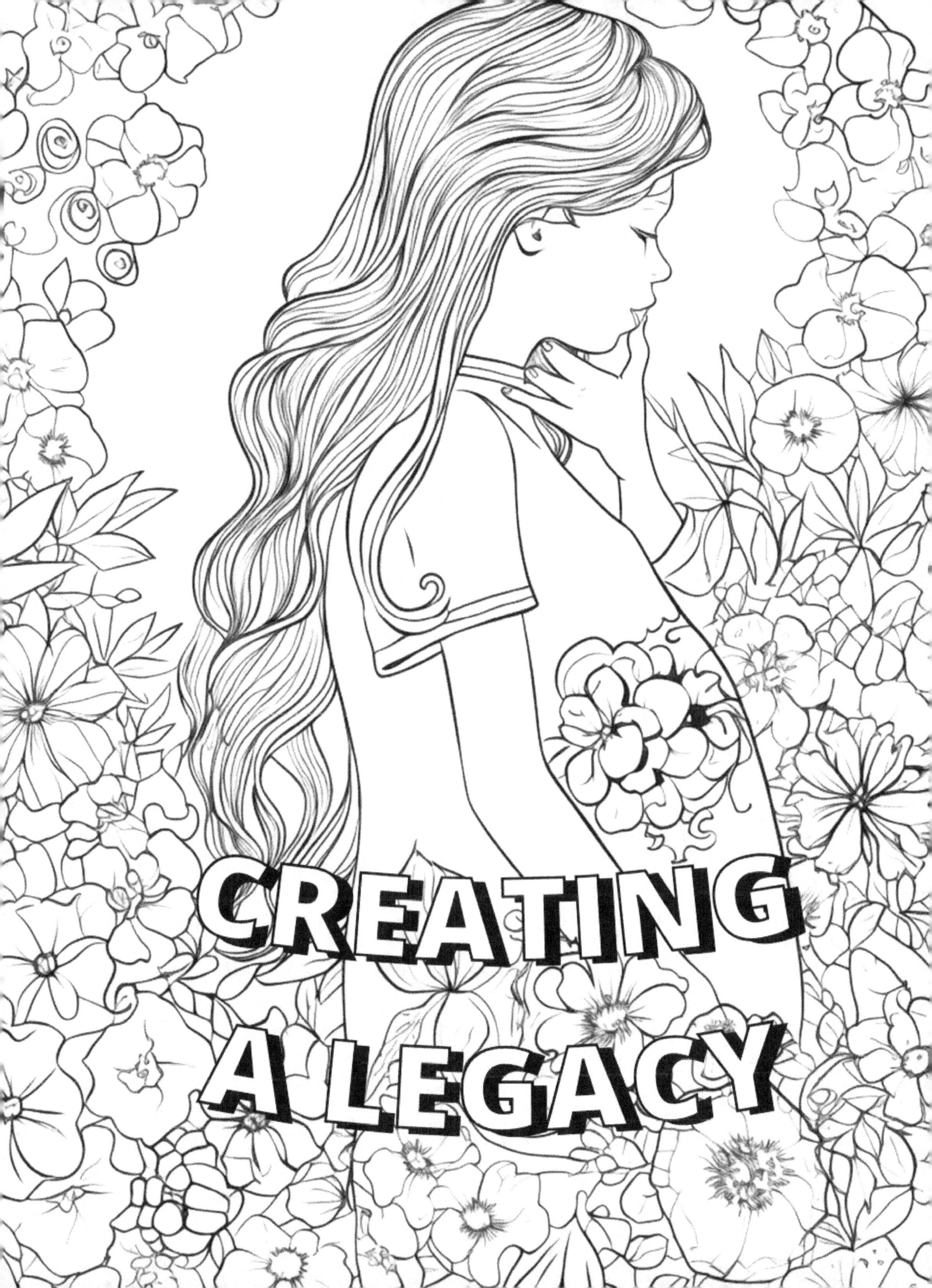
CREATING
A LEGACY

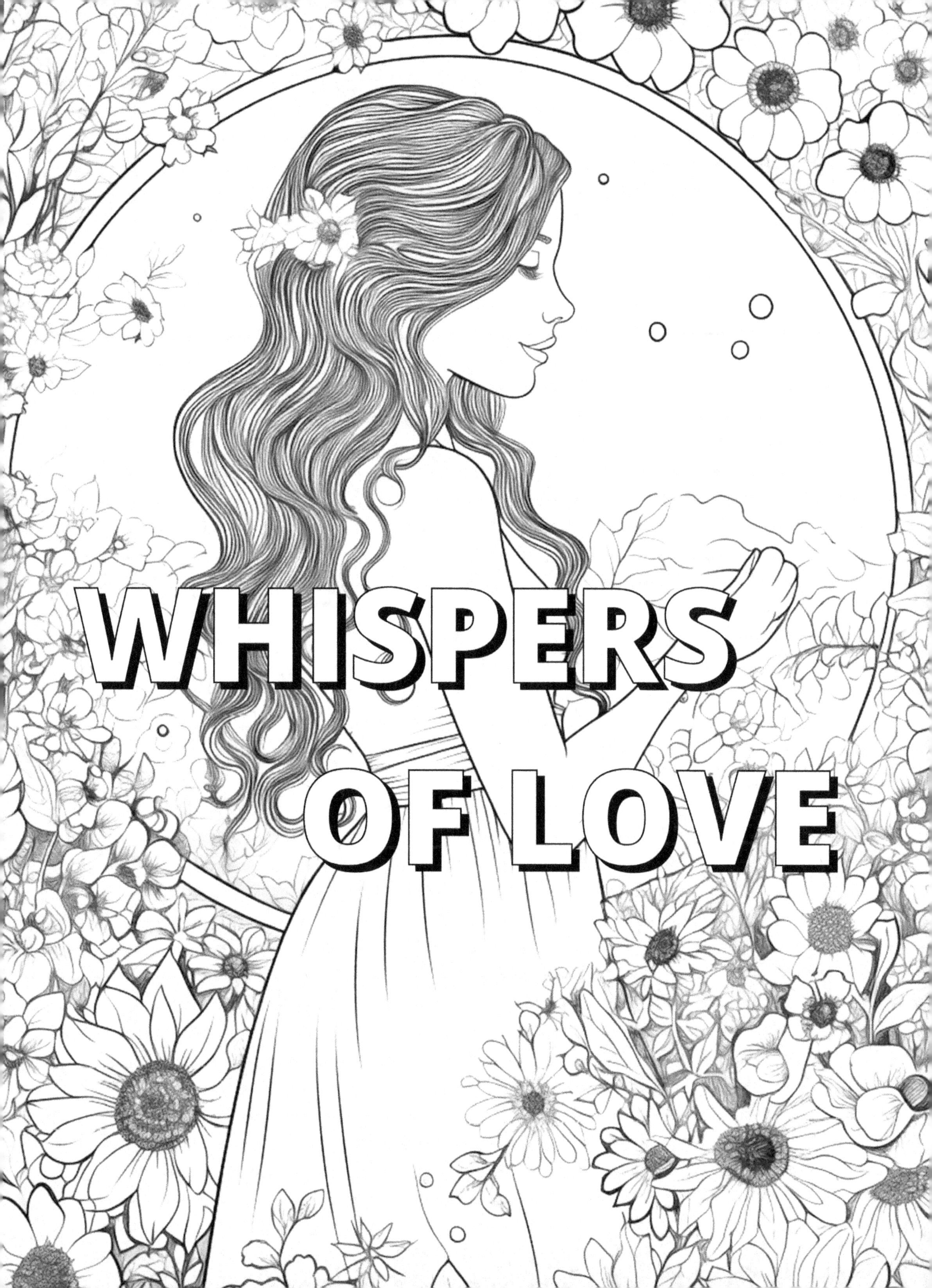

WHISPERS
OF LOVE

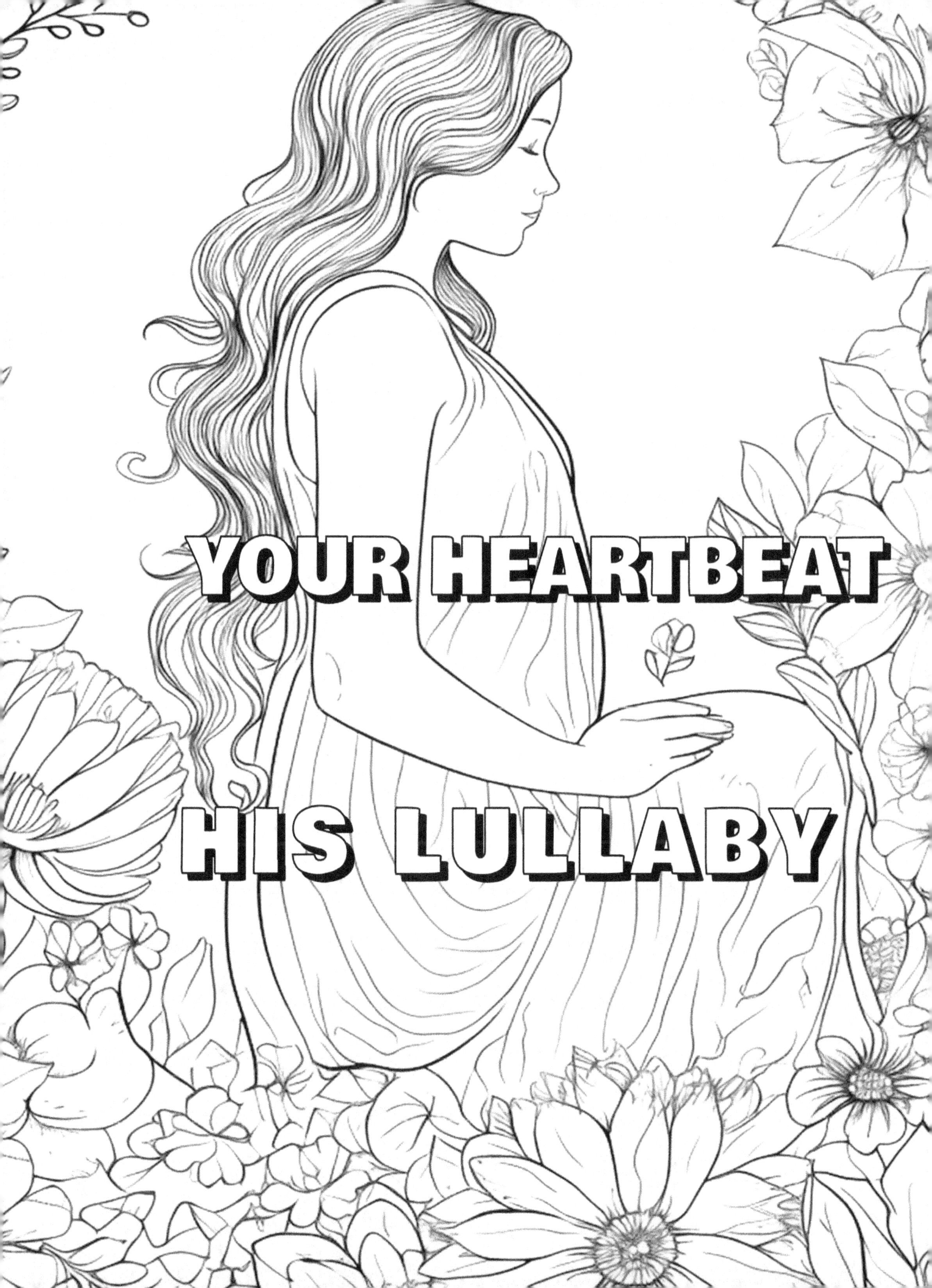

YOUR HEARTBEAT
HIS LULLABY

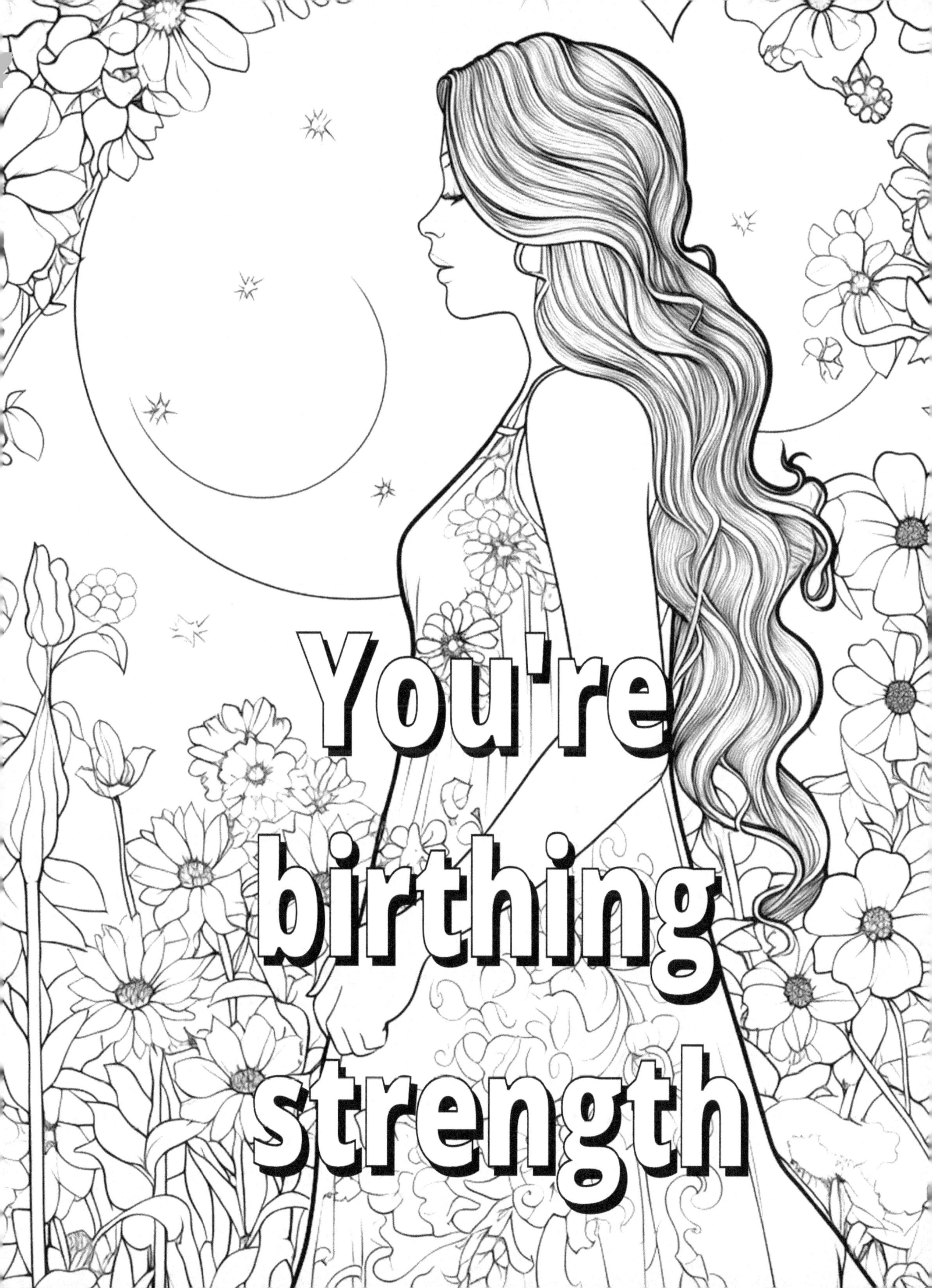
You're
birthing
strength

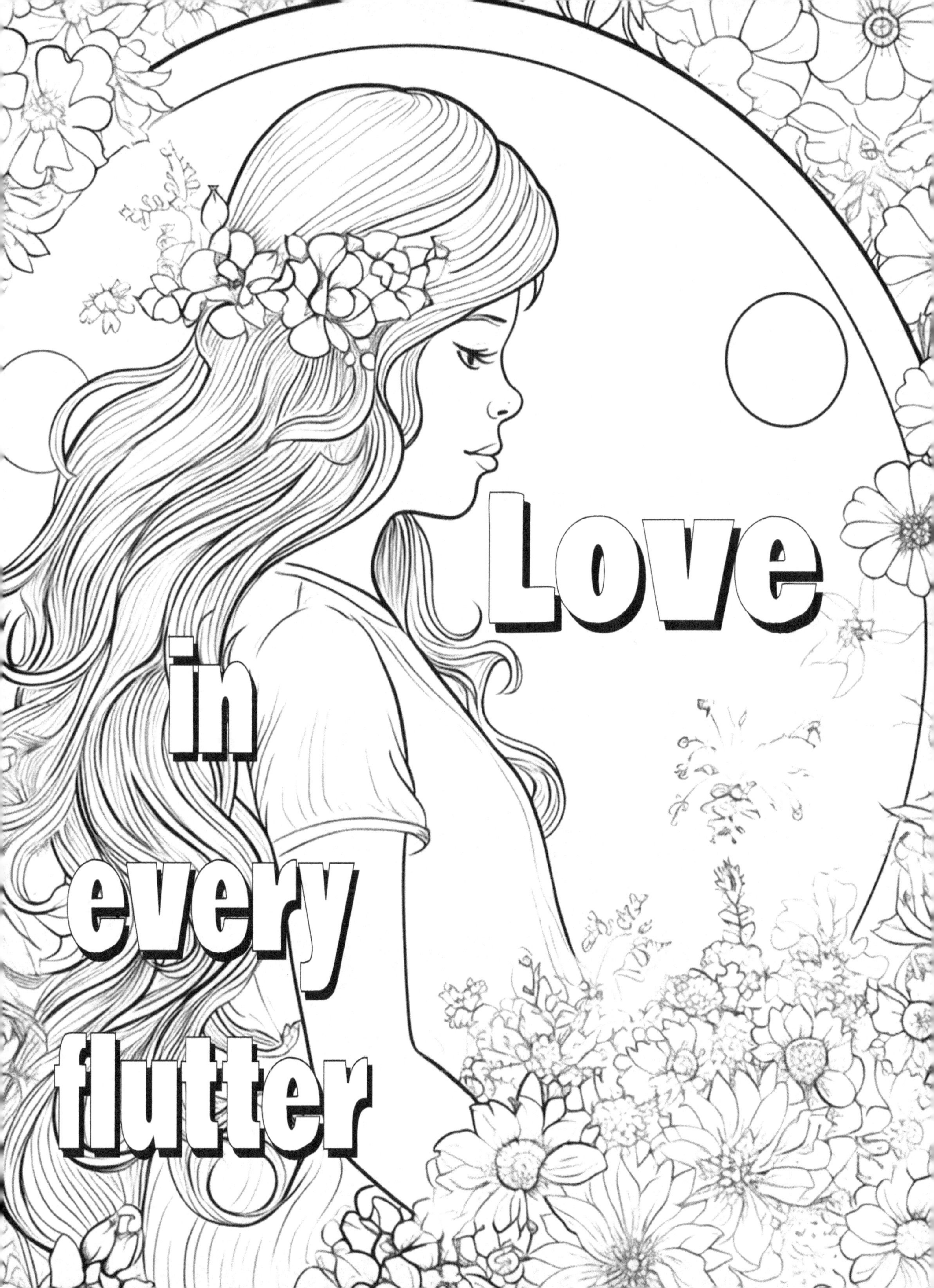

Love
in
every
flutter

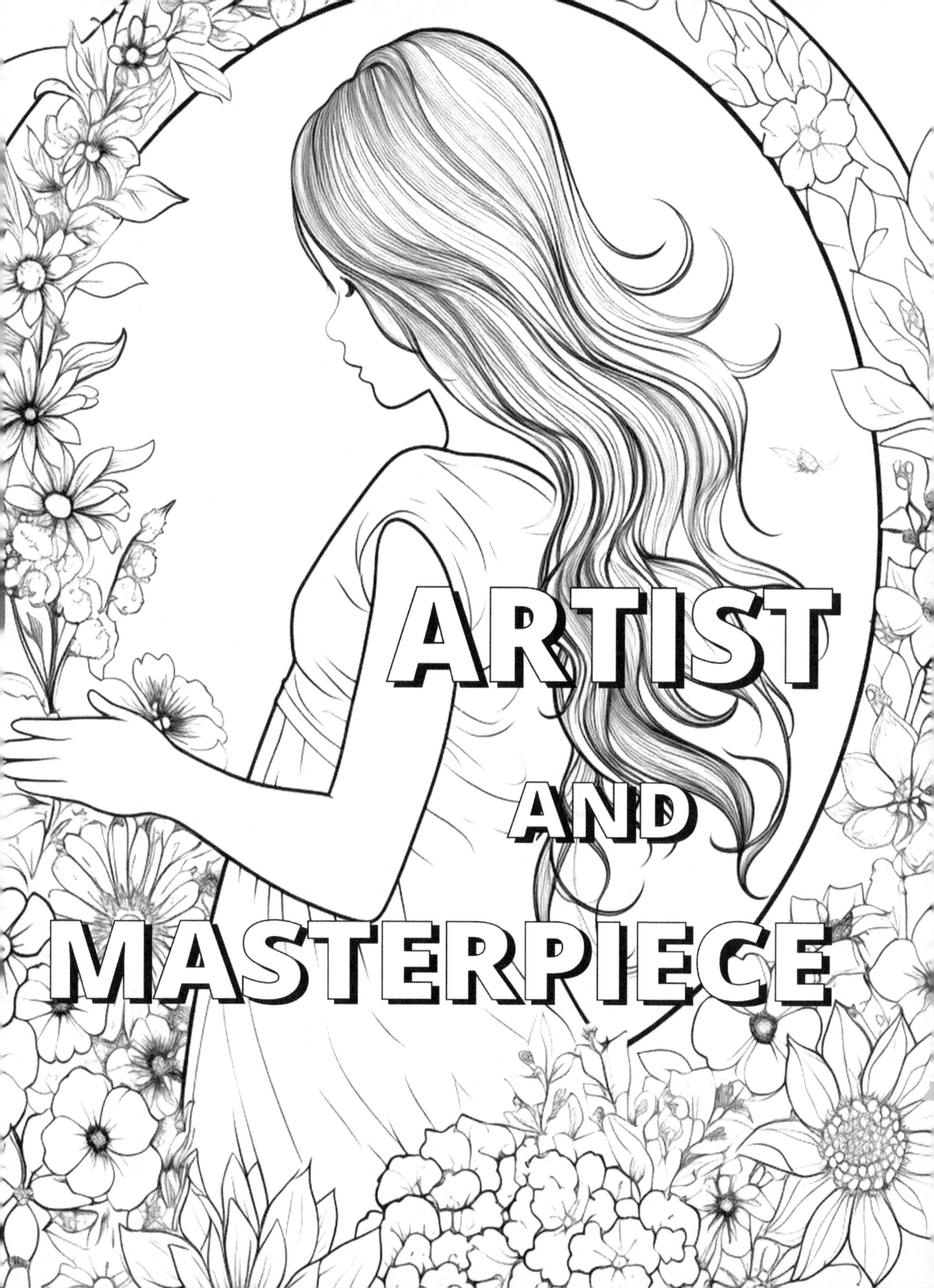

ARTIST
AND
MASTERPIECE

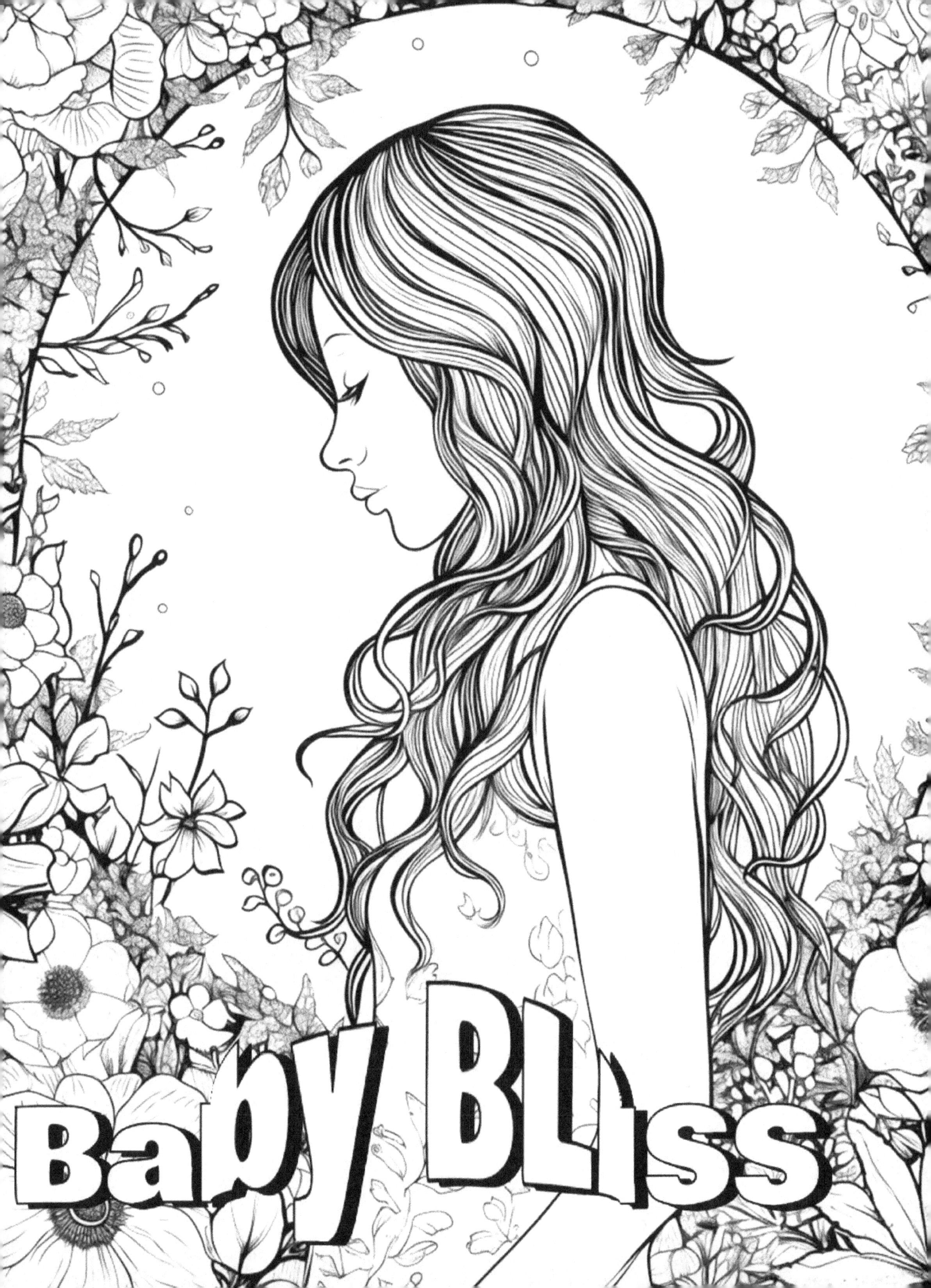

Baby Bliss

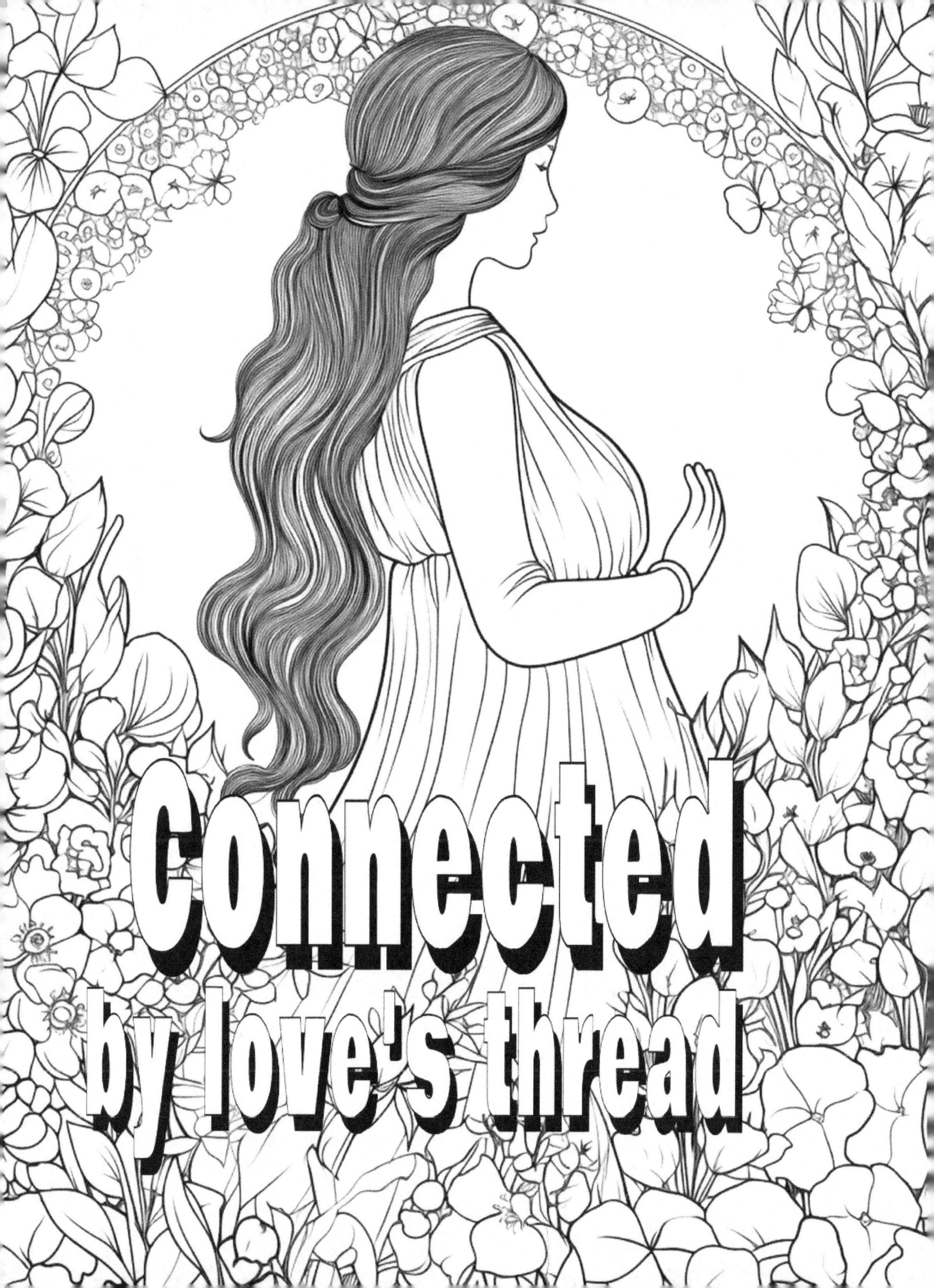

Connected
by love's thread

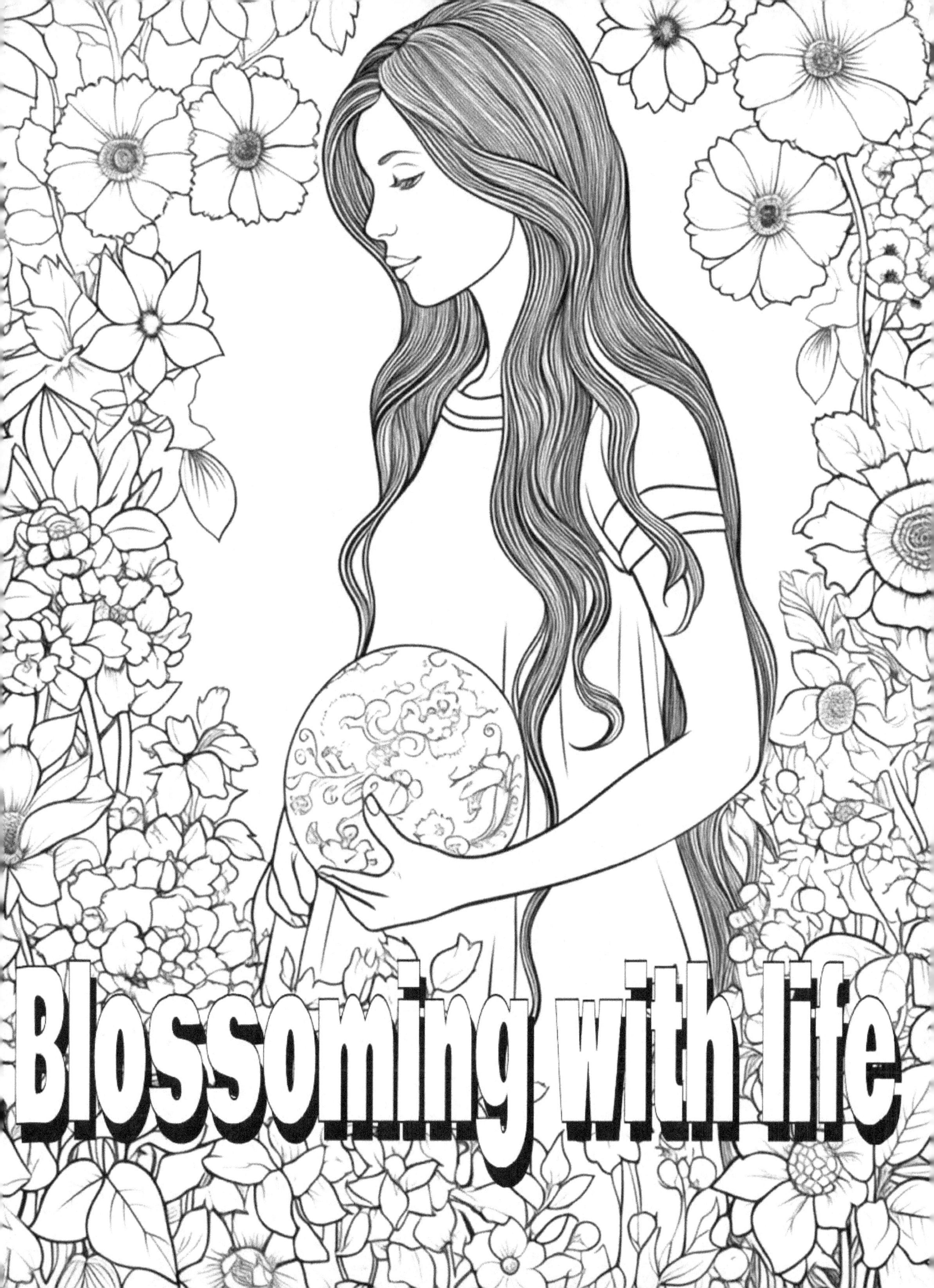
Blossoming with life

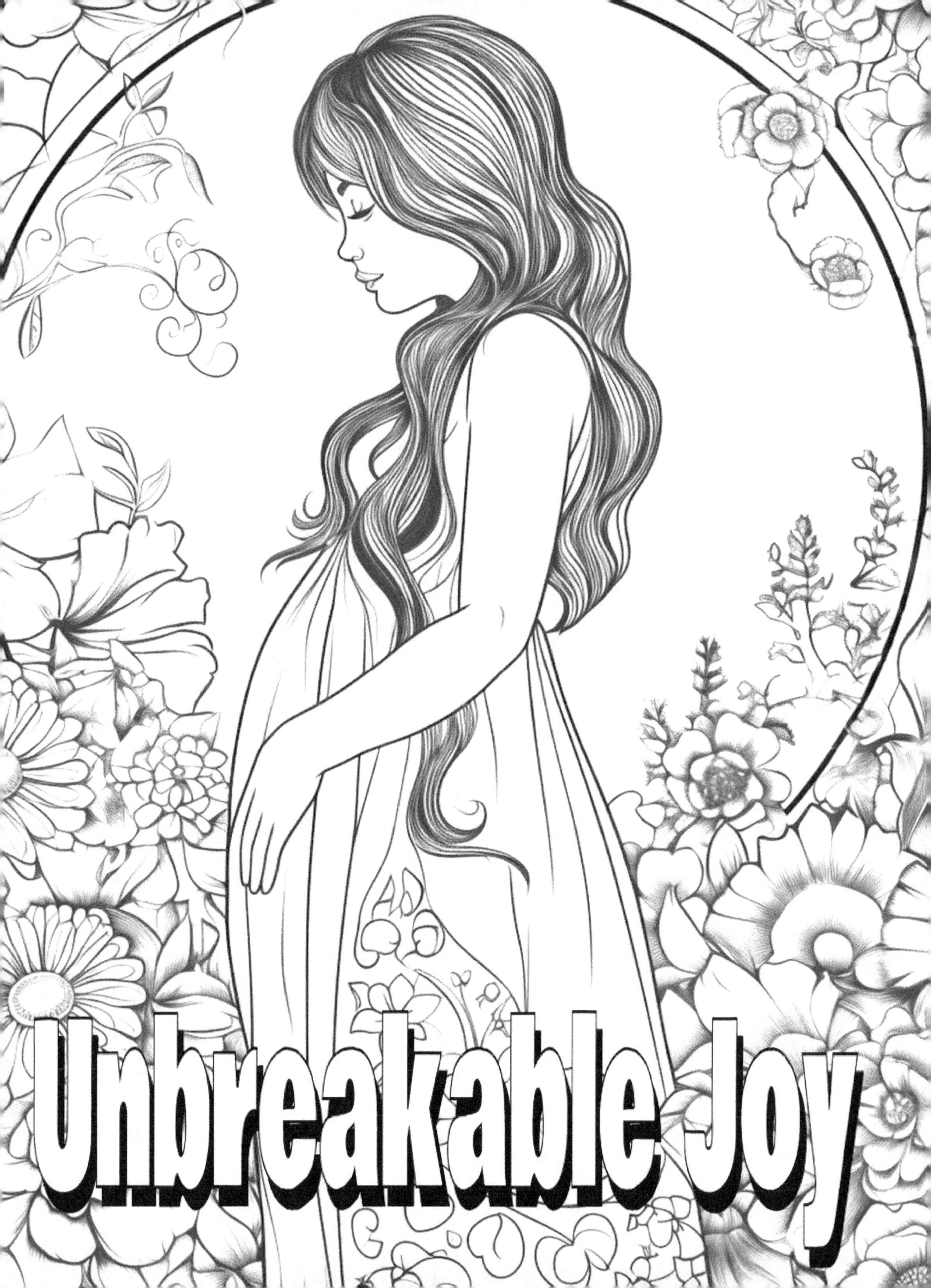
Unbreakable Joy

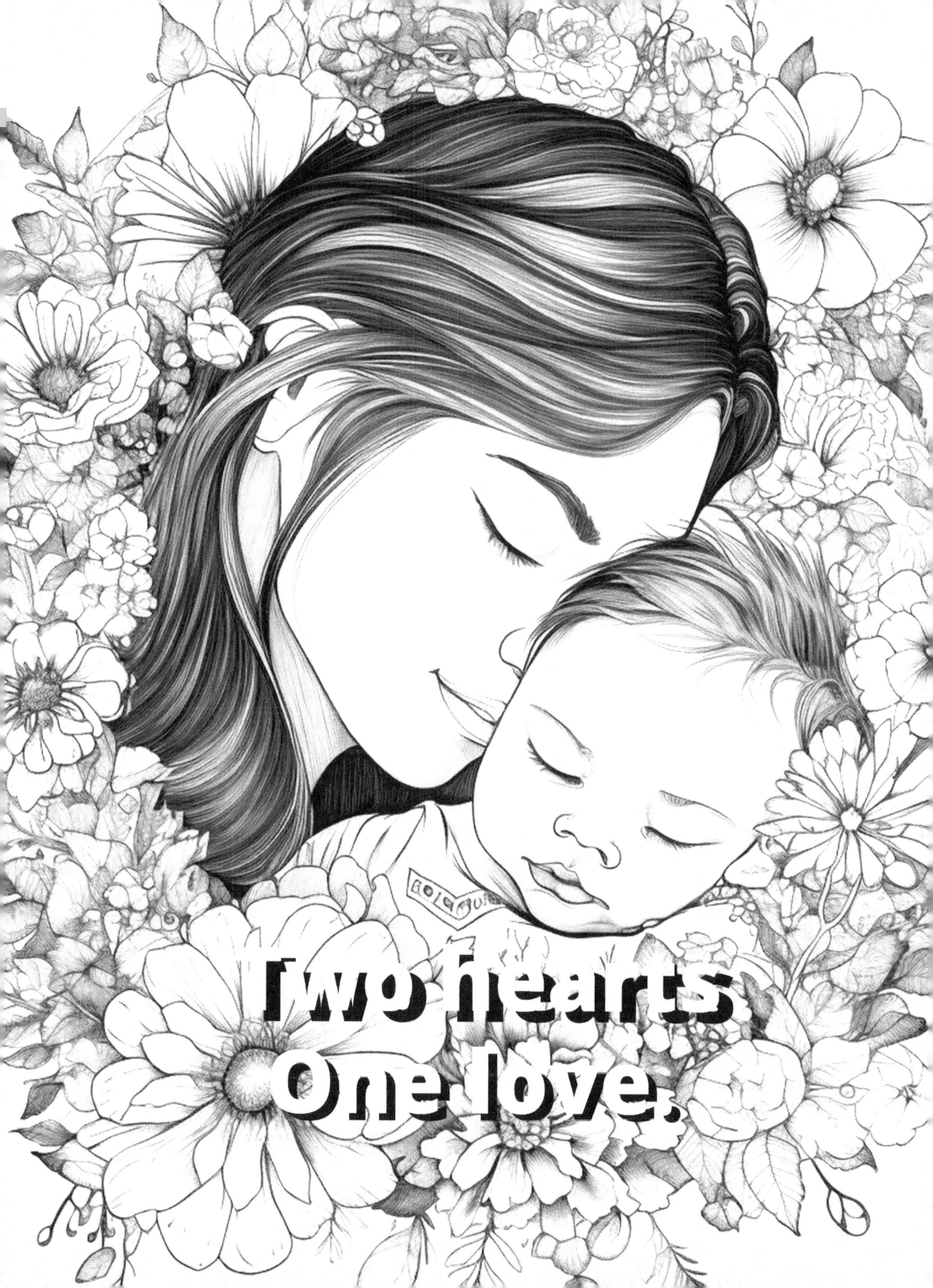
Two hearts
One love.